MW00685122

Combined Pharmacotherapy and Psychotherapy for Depression

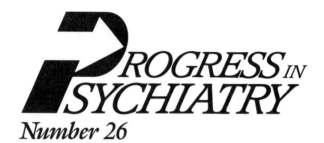

ROGRESS IN PSYCHIATRY

Number 26

David Spiegel, M.D.,
Series Editor

Combined Pharmacotherapy and Psychotherapy for Depression

Edited by
Donna W. Manning, M.D.
Allen J. Frances, M.D.

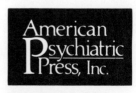

American Psychiatric Press, Inc.

Washington, DC
London, England

Note: The authors have worked to ensure that all information in this book concerning drug dosages, schedules, and routes of administration is accurate as of the time of publication and consistent with standards set by the U.S. Food and Drug Administration and the general medical community. As medical research and practice advance, however, therapeutic standards may change. For this reason and because human and mechanical errors sometimes occur, we recommend that readers follow the advice of a physician who is directly involved in their care or the care of a member of their family.

Books published by the American Psychiatric Press, Inc., represent the views and opinions of the individual authors and do not necessarily represent the policies and opinions of the Press or the American Psychiatric Association.

Copyright © 1990 American Psychiatric Press, Inc.
ALL RIGHTS RESERVED
Manufactured in the United States of America
First Edition   93 92 91 90   4 3 2 1

The paper used in this publication meets the minimum requirements of the American National Standard for Information Sciences — Permanence of Paper for Printed Library Materials, ANSI Z39.48-1984.   ∞

American Psychiatric Press, Inc.
1400 K Street, N.W.
Washington, DC 20005

Library of Congress Cataloging-in-Publication Data

Combined pharmacotherapy and psychotherapy for depression/edited by Donna W. Manning, Allen J. Frances. — 1st ed.
      p.   cm. — (Progress in psychiatry; no. 26)
   Includes bibliographical references.
   ISBN 0-88048-194-3 (alk. paper)
      1. Depression, Mental — Chemotherapy.
   2. Psychotherapy. 3. Combined modality therapy.
   I. Manning, Donna W., 1950–   . II. Frances, Allen,
   1942–   . III. Series.
      [DNLM: 1. Antidepressive Agents — therapeutic use.
   2. Combined Modality Therapy. 3. Depressive Disorder —
   therapy. 4. Psychotherapy. WM 171 C729]
   RC537.C635   1990
   616.85'2706 — dc20
   DNLM/DLC
   for Library of Congress   90-103
                                                           CIP

British Library Cataloguing in Publication Data

A CIP record is available from the British Library.

To my mother, Cynthia

D.M.

To my wife, Vera

A.F.

Contents

Contributors

Jules Bemporad, M.D.
Massachusetts Mental Health Center, Boston, Massachusetts

Lino Covi, M.D.
Johns Hopkins University, Baltimore, Maryland

Robert J. DeRubeis, Ph.D.
University of Pennsylvania, Philadelphia, Pennsylvania

Mark D. Evans, Ph.D.
University of Minnesota, Minneapolis, Minnesota

Allen J. Frances, M.D.
Cornell University Medical College, New York, New York

Ellen Frank, Ph.D.
University of Pittsburgh School of Medicine, and Western
Psychiatric Institute and Clinic, Pittsburgh, Pennsylvania

Steven D. Hollon, Ph.D.
Vanderbilt University, Nashville, Tennessee

Gerald L. Klerman, M.D.
Cornell University Medical College, New York, New York

David J. Kupfer, M.D.
University of Pittsburgh School of Medicine, Pittsburgh,
Pennsylvania

Janet Levenson, B.A.
University of Pittsburgh School of Medicine, and Western
Psychiatric Institute and Clinic, Pittsburgh, Pennsylvania

Ronald S. Lipman, Ph.D.
Friends Hospital, Philadelphia, Pennsylvania

Donna W. Manning, M.D.
Cornell University Medical College, New York, New York

Carl Salzman, M.D.
Massachusetts Mental Health Center, Boston, Massachusetts

James E. Smith II, M.D.
Johns Hopkins University, Baltimore, Maryland

Myrna M. Weissman, Ph.D.
Columbia University College of Physicians and Surgeons, New York, New York

Introduction to the Progress in Psychiatry Series

The Progress in Psychiatry Series is designed to capture in print the excitement that comes from assembling a diverse group of experts from various locations to examine in detail the newest information about a developing aspect of psychiatry. This series emerged as a collaboration between the American Psychiatric Association's (APA) Scientific Program Committee and the American Psychiatric Press, Inc. Great interest is generated by a number of the symposia presented each year at the APA annual meeting, and we realized that much of the information presented there, carefully assembled by people who are deeply immersed in a given area, would unfortunately not appear together in print. The symposia sessions at the annual meetings provide an unusual opportunity for experts who otherwise might not meet on the same platform to share their diverse viewpoints for a period of 3 hours. Some new themes are repeatedly reinforced and gain credence, while in other instances disagreements emerge, enabling the audience and now the reader to reach informed decisions about new directions in the field. The Progress in Psychiatry Series allows us to publish and capture some of the best of the symposia and thus provide an in-depth treatment of specific areas that might not otherwise be presented in broader review formats.

Psychiatry is by nature an interface discipline, combining the study of mind and brain, of individual and social environments, of the humane and the scientific. Therefore, progress in the field is rarely linear—it often comes from unexpected sources. Further, new developments emerge from an array of viewpoints that do not necessarily provide immediate agreement but rather expert examination of the issues. We intend to present innovative ideas and data that will enable you, the reader, to participate in this process.

We believe the Progress in Psychiatry Series will provide you with an opportunity to review timely new information in specific fields of interest as they are developing. We hope you find that the excitement of the presentations is captured in the written word and that this book proves to be informative and enjoyable reading.

David Spiegel, M.D.
Series Editor
Progress in Psychiatry Series

Progress in Psychiatry Series Titles

The Borderline: Current Empirical Research (#1)
Edited by Thomas H. McGlashan, M.D.

Premenstrual Syndrome: Current Findings and Future Directions (#2)
Edited by Howard J. Osofsky, M.D., Ph.D., and Susan J. Blumenthal, M.D.

Treatment of Affective Disorders in the Elderly (#3)
Edited by Charles A. Shamoian, M.D.

Post-Traumatic Stress Disorder in Children (#4)
Edited by Spencer Eth, M.D., and Robert S. Pynoos, M.D., M.P.H.

The Psychiatric Implications of Menstruation (#5)
Edited by Judith H. Gold, M.D., F.R.C.P.(C)

Can Schizophrenia Be Localized in the Brain? (#6)
Edited by Nancy C. Andreasen, M.D., Ph.D.

Medical Mimics of Psychiatric Disorders (#7)
Edited by Irl Extein, M.D., and Mark S. Gold, M.D.

Biopsychosocial Aspects of Bereavement (#8)
Edited by Sidney Zisook, M.D.

Psychiatric Pharmacosciences of Children and Adolescents (#9)
Edited by Charles Popper, M.D.

Psychobiology of Bulimia (#10)
Edited by James I. Hudson, M.D., and Harrison G. Pope, Jr., M.D.

Cerebral Hemisphere Function in Depression (#11)
Edited by Marcel Kinsbourne, M.D.

Eating Behavior in Eating Disorders (#12)
Edited by B. Timothy Walsh, M.D.

Tardive Dyskinesia: Biological Mechanisms and Clinical Aspects (#13)
Edited by Marion E. Wolf, M.D., and Aron D. Mosnaim, Ph.D.

Current Approaches to the Prediction of Violence (#14)
Edited by David A. Brizer, M.D., and Martha L. Crowner, M.D.

Treatment of Tricyclic-Resistant Depression (#15)
Edited by Irl L. Extein, M.D.

Introduction

A number of converging factors encouraged us to undertake this review of the combined use of psychotherapy and somatic therapy in the treatment of depression. Recent studies have made it clear that depression is a very commonly encountered problem both in randomly selected community populations and in psychiatry and medical practice. Depression is accompanied by serious morbidity and mortality. The presence of affective disorder is probably the strongest predictor of lifetime suicide risk, and many attempted and completed suicides occur in the midst of a clinical depression. Depression often results in serious inability to function interpersonally and intrapersonally.

It is fortunate that we now have available a variety of treatments with documented efficacy for depression. An extensive research literature has accumulated during the past 30 years on the treatment of depression with medication alone, and there is also a smaller and more recent literature on the treatment of depression with various forms of psychotherapy. The problem is now one of deciding which form of treatment or combination of treatments is most likely to be indicated in a given situation, made more complicated by the fact that the recent protocols governing either psychotherapy or drug studies usually must strive for purity and are thus necessarily restrictive of the additional therapies patients are permitted to receive. As a result, the pure treatments studied in research settings may not closely approximate those delivered in general clinical practice in which psychotherapy and antidepressant medication are often used together.

Fortunately, there are now enough studies that specifically set out to compare combined treatment with psychotherapy or drug therapy delivered alone that we can draw some early conclusions on the findings and perhaps more importantly can point out the methodological problems involved in such investigation. We can also benefit from the clinical experience that has been gained in combining medication with various types of psychotherapy in both acute and longer-term treatments.

There is a long history of the use of combined treatments for depression. As early as A.D. 30, Celsus laid down his prescription for melancholia, as it was then known, consisting of music to dissipate depressive cognitions and sedatives for insomnia coupled with a talking therapy in which "the patient is to be agreed with rather than opposed, and his mind slowly and imperceptibly is to be turned from irrational talk to something better. At times also his interest should be awakened" (Rosen 1968). Physicians in the Middle Ages recommended a variety of somatic treatments including purgatives, massage, exercise, and coitus along with "reassuring and gratifying measures to combat their suspicions, and pleasant and diverting conversations to lift their spirit."

Passage from the medieval period to the Renaissance saw continued use of the medicinal and verbal modes of therapy together. Robert Burton, in his treatise on melancholia, wrote: "First begin with prayer and then use physick; not one without the other but both together." He also advised seeking the support and distraction of a friend. A contemporary, Thomas Willis, described the need to "divert the soul from its troubling passions and cheering up the person," while administering purgatives, mineral water, and gentle hypnotics to combat sleeplessness (Jackson 1968).

The tendency to restrict treatments for depression to the somatic or the psychotherapeutic has a much more recent origin. This separation of approaches reflects what was an unfortunate and unnecessary split between biological and psychosocial psychiatry that occurred through much of this century. Although Freud was himself thoroughly biological in his understanding of psychopathology and predicted and would have undoubtedly welcomed somatic treatments, many of his followers tended toward a reductionistically nonbiological theoretical position in regard to pathogenesis and also maintained that somatic treatments would reduce a patient's motivation for change in psychotherapy. Biological clinicians often developed an equal reductionism of their own that ignored the psychosocial contributions to pathogenesis and risked a mechanistic delivery of medications in a fashion that reduced patient compliance and limited efficacy. The recent renewed interest in combined treatments reflects and promotes a more integrated view of psychopathology that recognizes multiple interacting causations and utilizes a variety of methods of observation.

Another trend that will become apparent has been the recent development of psychotherapeutic techniques that are specifically targeted to different aspects of depression. Most psychotherapy since the dawn of time has been relatively nonspecific and dependent for its effect on suggestion, positive expectancies, reversing demoralization, and offering a healing relationship. Even with the evolution of much more specific technical approaches in psychodynamic psychotherapy, the tendency was to treat different types of psychopathology with a broad-spectrum technique meant to be effective across a wide variety of diagnostic categories. Three factors have been prominent in promoting the more recent tendency to create specific psychotherapy techniques geared just for depression: 1) the development of reliable methods for diagnosing depression in a much more specific fashion, 2) the model of specificity offered by the somatic treatment for depression, and 3) the need in studies of psychotherapy outcome research for treatments that can be delivered in a standardized and replicative fashion.

Let us turn now to the contents of this book. It may be useful to introduce our authors and chapters and indicate what they are about. This volume begins in Chapter 1 with an overview of the research literature comparing the efficacy of combined drug and psychotherapy to either modality alone in the treatment of depression. We will critique and summarize the methodology and findings to date of this body of work. In Chapter 2, Drs. Hollon, DeRubeis, and Evans summarize the clinical and design considerations involved in conducting comparative outcome research with individual cognitive therapy and pharmacotherapy together versus each separately, with particular reference to their recently completed trial comparing imipramine treatment and individual cognitive therapy with the combination of the two. In Chapter 3, Drs. Covi, Lipman, and Smith discuss their work comparing group psychotherapy with and without drug treatment for depressed outpatients. We have placed their chapter in sequence after that of Drs. Hollon et al. because much of their work also involves the use of cognitive therapy. In Chapter 4, Drs. Weissman and Klerman summarize the nature and uses of interpersonal therapy in the treatment of depression both in combination with drug treatment and alone. Chapter 5 opens with a discussion by Drs. Frank and Kupfer and Ms. Levenson of the limited available research literature defining the role of combined pharmacotherapy and psychotherapy in the continuation and maintenance phases of the treatment of depression. They follow with a summary of their recently completed trial of the combination of interpersonal therapy and imipramine treatment versus each individually in the long-term management of depression. Chapter 6, by Drs. Salzman and Bemporad, rounds out our presentation with a clinician's perspective on the role of combined therapy in the treatment of depression. They elaborate their view that psychotherapy and pharmacotherapy work on distinct domains within the depressive syndrome, each acting to complement the efficacy of the other, and therefore are best used together in more severely depressed patients.

Before ending this introduction, we would like to acknowledge the important contributions made by Dr. Robert Prien to this area of research and to this book. Dr. Prien is head of the Somatic Treatments Section of the Affective and Anxiety Disorders Research Branch of the National Institute of Mental Health (NIMH). He has accomplished a great deal in promoting interest and research on the impact and indications for the combined treatment of depression. Most of the chapters presented here originated as presentations made to an NIMH workshop on the combined treatment of depression, which was organized by Dr. Prien and held in Washington, DC, 8–9 September 1987. A selection of these presentations also constituted a symposium held at the annual meeting of the American Psychiatric Association, 12 May 1988, in Montreal. Other individuals who contributed to the NIMH workshop and/or to the symposium and who helped to shape our thoughts on these issues include Drs. M. Tracie Shea, Robert Becker, Irene Elkin, Jan Fawcett, Robert Hirschfeld, Donald Klein, Marjorie Klein, Philip Lavori, George Murphy, Morris Parloff, Darrel Regier, and John Rush.

We would also like to acknowledge Dr. Michael H. Stone and Ms. Sylvia Erhart for their assistance in providing historical source material.

REFERENCES

Jackson SW: Melancholia and Depression. New Haven, CT, Yale University Press, 1968, pp 33, 59, 61, 97

Rosen G: Madness in Society. Chicago, IL, University of Chicago Press, 1968

Chapter 1

Combined Therapy for Depression: Critical Review of the Literature

Donna W. Manning, M.D.
Allen J. Frances, M.D.

Chapter 1

Combined Therapy for Depression: Critical Review of the Literature

Depressive disorders exact an enormous toll on the individual and society due to suicide, suffering, and impairment of job and family role functioning. The standard treatments for depression—psychotherapy and antidepressant medication—when administered individually each promote substantial improvement in only 60–80% of patients. Even among those who do respond to treatment, a substantial percentage do not experience full symptom remission nor are they necessarily protected from future recurrent depressive episodes. Furthermore, the onset of the therapeutic effect of medication or psychotherapy can be delayed for weeks to months from the start of treatment. Given these considerations, it is not surprising that the provision of a combination of psychotherapy and medication has become a widespread practice among clinicians who hope to achieve an additive, more complete, and more rapid effect than might result from either treatment delivered alone. Mirroring the interest among practitioners in combined therapy for depression, researchers have focused increasing attention in the last decade on clinical outcome trials comparing combined therapy in relation to single-component therapy.

Reviews summarizing the state of this research have proliferated in parallel with the studies themselves. Initial optimism as to the superiority of combined therapy relative to single-modality treatment has diminished in more recent reviews. Earlier reviews concluded that combined therapy is superior to either treatment delivered alone and found support for assertions that separate and specific effects of

We thank Ms. Sylvia Erhart for her invaluable research and editorial assistance in the preparation of this chapter.

pharmacotherapy and psychotherapy are discernible, suggesting an additive effect of the two modalities (Hollon and Beck 1978; Weissman 1979). More recent reviews draw more tempered conclusions, i.e., that combined therapy shows a modest superiority over either single component in some studies and may have a place in the treatment of selected patient populations such as those with severe depression and those with a history of poor response to single-modality therapy (Conte et al. 1986; Hollon and Beck 1978; Jarrett and Rush 1986; Shea et al. 1988; Weissman et al. 1987).

This review encompasses a literature of 17 combined therapy studies and, to our knowledge, is the most comprehensive that has been performed to date. In reviewing the literature, we asked several questions: How does combined therapy compare in efficacy to pharmacotherapy or psychotherapy alone in various outcome domains, e.g., vegetative symptoms, cognitive distortions, interpersonal functioning, time course of response, and selective effectiveness for depressive subgroups? If combined therapy is superior in efficacy to single-modality treatment, is this due to an enhanced or broader spectrum of effect? Are there specific combinations that are especially indicated or contraindicated? How trustworthy are the conclusions reached by existing studies, i.e., how methodologically sound are they?

METHODS

The 17 studies we included were compiled through a Medline search covering the years from 1969 to the present and through verbal communications with investigators in this area. Included are all English-language studies contrasting the combination of an anti-depressant drug and any specified form of psychotherapy with comparison conditions that included only one component of the combination as these were applied to patients with unipolar depression. Studies that did not adequately describe the treatments used or in which subject treatment assignment was nonrandom were excluded. Two such studies were found. In one (Teasdale et al. 1984), in which patients treated for depression by general practitioners were randomized to cognitive therapy versus no additional treatment, the study authors did not adequately define treatment received. In the second report (Beutler et al. 1987), which compared the combination of group cognitive therapy and alprazolam with each treatment alone, cell assignment was nonrandom. We did not require that a placebo control be included.

We used the box-score method of aggregating studies, which requires the categorization of each study as to whether combined therapy is more, less, or equally effective than a given comparison treatment. Totals across studies for each of the three possible outcomes are then tallied. A major limitation of this approach is that it requires the literature reviewer to make difficult judgment calls on study results that are frequently open to alternative interpretation. For example, combined therapy may be superior to the comparison condition on one very important outcome variable while only comparable in other less important ones; or the therapy may be superior on some measures and inferior on others. The box-score method is more quantitative than the narrative method used in most previous reviews of this literature. It is, however, far less precise than a metanalysis, which takes into account the relative differences in methodological soundness of each study and utilizes the effect size, a statistic that allows for the aggregation of raw data from various studies and its transformation into a common metric. Our literature review did not use metanalytic methods because the raw data reported in studies provides insufficient information and is often deficient in providing standard deviations and/or the results of direct cell comparisons. This lack in the current reporting of data should provide a caution for investigators in future reports. If we are eventually to have a literature that lends itself to convenient aggregation, it is crucial that reports provide adequate raw data and suitable between-group comparisons.

DESCRIPTIVE OVERVIEW OF THE LITERATURE

Table 1-1 provides an indication of the rate of accumulation of studies and their types over time. Until 1974, only one controlled study on the combined treatment of depression had appeared in the literature (Daneman 1961). Since that time, reports have been published at an accelerating rate. Early studies compared psychodynamic therapies in combination with drug therapies, whereas from 1974 to 1980,

Table 1-1. Study treatments as a function of time

Therapy	1960–1969	1970–1979	1980–present
Psychodynamic	1	1	0
Marital	0	1	0
Behavior	0	0	4
Interpersonal	0	2	2
Cognitive	0	0	6
Total	1	4	12

interpersonal therapy was the predominant mode of therapy investigated. From 1980 on, cognitive-behavior therapy has been the most
frequently used therapy component in combination studies. Although
the majority of studies used an individual-therapy format, a few have
looked at group and marital treatment combined with medication.

The treatment conditions or cells contrasted with combined
therapy have varied considerably among studies. As outlined by
Hollon and DeRubeis (1981), there are eight possible comparison
conditions: psychotherapy alone or in combination with placebo,
pharmacotherapy alone or coupled with sham psychotherapy, placebo
and sham therapy alone or together, and no treatment at all (Table
1-2). The most frequent type of comparison between cells has been
between combined therapy versus psychotherapy or psychotherapy
and placebo (24 of 41 studies). Combined therapy was compared with
drug treatment alone or drug treatment with attention control only
half as often (11 of 41 studies). This may reflect the interest of the
investigators in psychotherapy. It is our observation that none of the
studies were conducted by investigators whose primary interest is in
psychopharmacology. Cognitive therapy was the most frequently
investigated therapy (6 studies), followed closely by interpersonal
therapy and behavior therapy with 4 studies each, psychodynamic
therapy with only 2 studies, and marital therapy with 1 study. This
frequency distribution probably does not mirror general clinical
practice in which psychodynamic treatments continue to pre-
dominate, but until recently, these have been more difficult to study
systematically.

The drugs most often used in combination studies have been
amitriptyline (6 studies) and imipramine (5 studies). It is of great
interest that there are only 7 studies providing a placebo condition in
comparison with the combined conditions. This makes it difficult to
rule out that any superior efficacy of the combined conditions is not
simply a function of an augmented placebo effect.

The number of subjects enrolled in studies varied greatly (Table
1-3). Although many patients were often enrolled in these studies,
the large number of cells included in the study designs resulted in an
average of only 26 patients per treatment cell. Only two studies had
more than 30 patients per cell, which is likely to be the minimum
number required to achieve adequate statistical power to detect the
small (but potentially significant) differences that combined treatments may bring to augment what are already effective antidepressant
treatments (Cohen 1969).

The preponderance (15 of 17) of studies listed in Table 1-4 focused
on the acute phase of the treatment of depression. Half of the studies
included a follow-up (Table 1-5), whereas only 4 looked at the

Table 1-2. Treatment comparisons

	Drug and dynamic	Drug and marital	Drug and behavior	Drug and interpersonal	Drug and cognitive	Total
Drug alone	0	0	1	2	2	5
Therapy alone	1	0	1	2	8	12
Therapy plus placebo	2	1	5	3	1	12
Drug plus attention control	2	1	1	1	1	6
Attention control plus placebo	1	1	0	1	0	3
Attention control alone	0	0	0	1	0	1
Placebo alone	0	0	0	1	0	1
No treatment	0	0	0	1	0	1
Total	6	3	8	12	12	41

Table 1-3. Summary of study characteristics

Variable	Mean	Range	Number of studies reporting ($N = 17$)
Sample size	91	18–230	17
n per cell	26	6–55[a]	14
Sample demographics			
Sex (% female)	76	44–100	17
Age (years)	42(37)[b]	17–81	15
Education (years)	12	11–16	12
% married	50	10–74	12
% employed	58	39–81	8
Race (% white)	88	77–100	9
Profile of depressive symptoms			
Duration of episode (months)		3–50	8
% RDC probable or definite endogenous	57	32–91	5
% situational	53	27–76	4
% with previous episode	56	22–76	8
HRSD score		18–25	5
BDI score		24–30	4
Study parameters			
Phase of treatment studied			
Acute			15
Continuation			3
Maintenance			1
Follow-up			7
Length (weeks)			
Acute-treatment phase	13	7–20	16
Total treatment phase	24	6–156	16
Treatment and follow-up	47	6–164	16
No. of treatment cells	3.5	2–6	17
No. of therapy sessions (acute)	16	7–30	15
Antidepressant medication			
Tricyclic			14
Other (MAOI, lithium, benzodiazepine ± TCA)			3
TCA dose (mg/dl)	179	100–300	10
Duration of medication treatment (weeks) (acute phase)	14	6–20	17

Note. RDC = Research Diagnostic Criteria. HRSD = Hamilton Rating Scale for Depression. BDI = Beck Depression Inventory. MAOI = monoamine oxidase inhibitor. TCA = tricyclic antidepressant.
[a]Only two studies had ≥30 patients/cell.
[b]No. in parentheses excludes geriatric studies.

Table 1-4. Summary of combined therapy studies: acute treatment

Study	Patient characteristics	Cells	Treatment variables Psychotherapy	Pharmacotherapy	Weeks of treatment	Results	Comments
Daneman 1961	195 (69% female), ages 17–75 Subtypes: 82% neurotic 16% psychotic 2% organic	C Pd	Individual psychoanalytically oriented therapy 1–2 times/wk	IMI 50–200 mg/day (mean 100)	9–12	C > Pd	Patients allowed to engage in therapy outside of protocol; therapist also served as rater
Covi et al. 1974	149 female, ages 20–50 (mean age 34) with chronic depression	C D_1p D_2p Pd cpd	Psychoanalytically oriented group, 90 min/wk *Placebo:* brief supportive psychotherapy 20 min every 2 wk	D_1: IMI 100–200 mg/day (mean 150) D_2: Diazepam 10–20 mg/day (mean 15)	16	C = D_1p C > Pd IMI > diazepam No differences between completer and end-point results	Only 2 therapists; high attrition
Friedman 1975	196 (79% female), ages 21–67 Subtypes: 88% neurotic 8% psychotic 2% bipolar	C Dp Pd cpd	Conjoint marital therapy, 1 time/wk *Placebo:* 7 half-hour structured sessions	AMI 100–200 mg/day	12	C = Dp = Pd = cpd: marital therapy has late effect to improve family relations; AMI reduces depressive symptoms early on	Diagnostic heterogeneity; limited test reliability data; patients included in analysis who never returned for evaluation; no direct comparison of treatment cells; raters not blind to treatment.

Table 1-4. Summary of combined therapy studies: acute treatment—Continued

Study	Patient characteristics	Cells	Treatment variables		Weeks of treatment	Results	Comments
			Psychotherapy	Pharmacotherapy			
DiMascio et al. 1979 Weissman et al. 1979 Prusoff et al. 1980 Weissman et al. 1981 Rounsaville et al. 1981	96 (86% female)	C D P p	Interpersonal therapy, 1 time/wk *Placebo:* nonscheduled treatment—patients told to contact therapist whenever they felt need; ≤1 session/mo	AMI 100–200 mg/day	16	Completers: C = D = P = p End point: C > all other conditions Situational depression: C = P = D Endogenous depression: C > all other conditions	Selective sample (all nonresponders to D or P over last 3 mo excluded)
Wilson 1982	64 (66% female), ages 20–55, recruited from ads	C Dp Pd cpd	Task assignment or relaxation training 1 session/wk *Placebo:* two 1-hour unstructured sessions	AMI 150 mg/day for 6 wk	7	C = Dp = Pd = cpd	Inexperienced therapists; inflexible drug schedule; use of nonstandard outcome measures; short duration of treatment
Roth et al. 1982	26 (66% female), ages 24–47, recruited from ads	C P	Self-control group therapy, 2-hour sessions, 1 session/wk	DMI 150 or 200 mg/day	12	C = P in degree of symptom reduction and self-control variables; C > P in rate of symptom reduction	Inexperienced therapists; small N

Study	Sample	Groups	Treatment	Medication	No.	Results	Comments
Murphy et al. 1984	80 (77% female)	C Pd D P	Cognitive therapy—2 sessions/wk for 8 wk then 1/wk for 4 wk	Nortriptyline dosage adjusted to blood level *Placebo*: atropine, phenobarbital	12	$C = D = P = Pd$ in reducing depressive symptoms; $C + P + Pd > D$ in maintaining patients with BDI score ≤ 4; No completer/endpoint differences	Used well-tolerated medication and blood levels; duration of medication flexible; number of sessions controlled at 20
Beck et al. 1985	33 (72% female)	C P	Cognitive therapy, 20 sessions	AMI 75–200 mg/day (mean 152)	12	$C = P$	Small cell size; no blinding; inexperienced therapist; TCA poorly tolerated, limiting dosage
Covi and Lipman 1987	70 (60% female), mean age 44	C_1 P_1 P_2	P_1: group cognitive-behavior therapy; P_2: interpersonal/dynamic group—2-hour sessions 1–2 times/wk + 3 individual sessions (4 booster sessions given to nonimproved patients)	IMI 50–300 mg/day (mean 135–185)	14	$C_1 = P_1 > P_2$ in reducing depressive and anxiety symptoms; $C_1 > P_1$ or P_2 in reducing phobic anxiety and somatization	Overall, well-designed study; only 2 therapists; high attrition

Table 1-4. Summary of combined therapy studies: acute treatment—Continued

Study	Patient characteristics	Cells	Treatment variables		Weeks of treatment	Results	Comments
			Psychotherapy	Pharmacotherapy			
Rush and Watkins 1981	44 (86% female)	C_1 P_1 P_2	P_1: individual cognitive therapy; P_2: group cognitive therapy—maximum of 20 sessions (mean of 15)	AMI, doxepin 150 mg/day; phenylzine 60–90 mg/day; Lithium adjusted to blood level 0.8–1.2 meq	10–12	P_1 and $C_1 > P_2$; $P_1 = C_1$; C_1 and P_1 produce similar response patterns; Significant differences between cells in mean no. of sessions; No difference between completer and end-point results	Small cell sizes; 3 ADs used; P cell patients allowed to be on psychotropic medication; weak statistics; patients not randomly assigned; some patients in P_2 cells on psychotropic medication
Blackburn and Bishop 1983 Blackburn et al. 1981	GP: 24 (80% female) OPD: 40 (75% female) Both groups ages 18–25	C D P	Both samples: cognitive therapy 1–2 sessions/wk for 3 wk; then 1/wk for a maximum of 20 wk	AMI or CMI $\geq$ 150 mg/day, given by GP to GP sample and by psychiatrist to OPD sample	20	GP: C = P > D on depressive and cognitive variables; OPD: C > P > D on depressive and cognitive variables	No blinding; no independent rating after baseline; small cell size; GPs administered drug in GP sample
Bellack et al. 1981, 1983 Hersen et al. 1984	125 females, ages 21–60 (mean age 30); chronic	C_1 P_1d P_2d D	P_1: social skills training P_2: time-limited dynamic therapy—acute: 1 session/wk for 12 wk; continuation: 6–8 sessions over 6 mo	AMI 50–300 mg/day (acute mean 178)	12	Overall outcome: $C_1 = P_1d = P_2d = D$; Social skills measures: social skills training with or without drugs was superior	Significant differences between cells in attrition rates

Study	Sample	Conditions	Treatment	Medication	N	Results	Comments
Rothblum et al. 1982	18 (72% female), ages 61–81, recruited from ads	C_1 C_2 Pd	Interpersonal therapy 1 session/wk	D_1: Alprazolam D_2: IMI ? dosage	6	Preliminary: compliance and response to treatment were comparable with younger patients	High percentage of patients screened could not be included in study due to medical problems, etc.; small sample size
Becker and Heimberg 1987	39 (48% female), mean age 39	C_1 C_2 P_1d P_2d	P_1: social skills training P_2: crises supportive therapy 1 session/wk for 16 wk then bi-weekly for 4 wk	Nortriptyline adjusted to blood level	20	Preliminary: all treatments effective; $C_1 = P_1d = C_2 = P_2d$ on all but 2 measures	No placebo + attention control condition
Hollon and Najavits 1988	106, mean age 34	C D P	Cognitive therapy, maximum of 20 sessions	IMI 200–300 mg/day for 12 wk; blood level 180 mg/ml	12	Acute treatment: C > D, C > P, D = P, on measures of depression; no difference between completer and end-point data using estimated end-point analysis	Overall, well-designed study: high attrition and consequent small cell size

Note. C = combined therapy. D = pharmacotherapy. P = psychotherapy alone. d = placebo only. p = attention control. Dp = pharmacotherapy plus attention control. Pd = psychotherapy plus placebo. cpd = attention control plus placebo. IMI = imipramine. AMI = amitripyline. DMI = desipramine. BDI = Beck Depression Inventory. TCA = tricyclic antidepressant. ADs = antidepressants. OPD = outpatient clinic. CMI = clomipramine. GP = general practice.

Table 1-5. Studies including follow-up data

Study	Patient charac- teristics	Cells	Treatment variables		Months of treatment	Follow-up methods	Results	Comments
			Psychotherapy	Pharmacotherapy				
Weissman et al. 1981	62	C D P P	Interpersonal therapy	AMI	12	Retrospective monthly ac- counts of treat- ment in follow- up period	C = D = P = p in type and amount of treat- ment received and depressive indices; interper- sonal therapy > D on social functioning	Retrospective data collection
Roth et al. 1982	26	C P	Self-control therapy	DMI	3	BDI	Treatment gains maintained; C = P	Small *N*
Wilson 1982	52	C Dp Pd cpd	Task assign- ment and relaxation training	AMI	6	Self ratings monthly; investi- gator rating at 6 mo	C = Dp = Pd = cpd; main ef- fect of therapy to reduce need for reentry into treatment	
Beck et al. 1985	33	C P	Cognitive therapy	AMI	12	BDI and HRSD at 6 and 12 mo	C = P at 6 and 12 mo. P > C in no. of follow-up therapy sessions	Small *N*

Study	N	Group	Therapy	Drug	Duration	Measures	Outcome	Comments
Simons et al. 1986 Murphy et al. 1984	44 responders	C Pd D P	Cognitive therapy	Nortriptyline	12	Several rating scales administered at 1, 6, and 12 mo	C = P = Pd = D; trend for therapy to prophylax against relapse	
Blackburn et al. 1986 Blackburn et al. 1981	41 responders	C D P	Cognitive therapy	AMI/ CMI	24	HRSD, BDI at 6 mo; case records monitored at 6, 12, 18, and 24 mo	C = P > D in reducing risk of recurrence or relapse at 2 yr	Use of return to M.D. for treatment as measure of relapse or recurrence may underestimate poor outcome
Evans et al. 1985	43 responders	C D_1 D_2 P	Cognitive therapy	D_1: IMI 200–300 mg/day for 12 wk D_2: IMI ≤ acute dose for 1 yr	24	BDI, life events report monthly; investigator rating every 6 mo	C = P = D_2 > D_1 in reducing relapses/recurrence	

Note. C = combined therapy. D = pharmacotherapy alone. P = psychotherapy alone. d = placebo only. p = attention control. Dp = pharmacotherapy plus attention control. Pd = psychotherapy plus placebo. cpd = attention control plus placebo. AMI = amitriptyline. DMI = desipramine. BDI = Beck Depression Inventory. HRSD = Hamilton Rating Scale for Depression. CMI = clomipramine. IMI = imipramine.

continuation or maintenance phases (Table 1-6). The overwhelming emphasis on treatment effects for the index period of depression does not address the issue of relative durability of treatment effect of combined versus individual therapy in what is often a recurring illness.

Almost all the studies we reviewed utilized the Hamilton Rating Scale for Depression (HRSD) (Hamilton 1967) and the Beck Depression Inventory (BDI) (Beck 1978). Additional instruments used reflected the theoretical underpinnings of the psychotherapists employed such that studies of cognitive-behavior therapy emphasized measures of change in depressive cognitions, whereas interpersonal therapy studies emphasized indices of change in social and role functioning. Unfortunately, aside from the HRSD and the BDI, there was little overlap in outcome measures between studies, making it difficult to assess the results in a cumulative way on other instruments.

METHODOLOGICAL LIMITATIONS

A number of methodological problems confound the literature on combined therapy and make this a particularly difficult research subject. For instance, several studies measured combined therapy against a given psychotherapy at a center known for its allegiance to that psychotherapeutic approach, thereby introducing the potential for bias in both the investigator and the subjects. Subject selection poses another problem in that the need for a homogeneous population with respect to demographic and symptomatic characteristics may well have resulted in the inclusion of so small a percentage of subjects initially screened as to severely limit generalizability to the population at large.

The shortcoming that most hampers the interpretation of the available literature is the relatively small number of subjects completing the protocols. This limits the statistical power to protect against Type II errors of finding no difference when a difference does indeed exist. This is a special concern in this type of research because the combined treatment must compete with what have already been demonstrated to be quite effective treatments delivered alone. This provides little room at the top for showing additional effects and requires larger sample sizes and the use of a wider array of outcome measures to provide additional room for finding variance.

There are several issues relevant to the selection and structuring of treatment conditions that also limit the interpretation of results. Most striking may be the lack of comparison between active treatment and placebo and/or attention control conditions. For instance, it is not yet clearly established that antidepressant drug therapy is more effective than placebo in alleviating the mild to moderate range of depres-

Table 1-6. Studies including a continuation or maintenance treatment phase

Study	Patient characteristics	Cells	Psychotherapy	Pharmacotherapy treatment	Months of treatment	Results	Comments
Klerman et al. 1974 Weissman et al. 1974 Paykel et al. 1975	150 female, ages 20–60 (mean age 39)	C Dp P Pd P cpd	Individual interpersonal therapy 1 time/ wk *Placebo:* 1 session/mo for prescribing and/or assessment	AMI 100– 150 mg/ day	8	Interpersonal therapy improved social functioning; AMI reduced relapse rate; C offers no advantage over P or D alone	Only TCA responders selected; only study with 6-cell design; no direct cell comparisons
Blackburn et al. 1981 Blackburn and Bishop 1983	41 responders from acute study	C D P	Cognitive therapy booster sessions every 6 wk	AMI/CMI at acute or reduced dose	6	$C = P = D$ on mean symptom scores, C and C + P analyzed together > D in reducing rate of recurrence	
Hersen et al. 1984	125	C_1 P_1d P_2d D	P_1: social skills training P_2: time-limited dynamic therapy 6–8 sessions	AMI 150 mg/day (mean 163)	6	$C_1 = P_1d = P_2d = D$; social skills training improves scores of social functioning	

Table 1-6. Studies including a continuation or maintenance treatment phase—Continued

Study	Patient characteristics	Cells	Treatment variables		Months of Pharmacotherapy treatment	Results	Comments
			Psychotherapy	Pharmacotherapy			
Frank and Kupfer 1987	128 (77% female) (mean age 39), recurrently depressed responders to acute- and continuous-phase interpersonal therapy and IMI	C Pd Dp P cpd	Maintenance interpersonal therapy: monthly sessions	IMI 150–300 mg/day	36	Results in press	Author notes difficulty distinguishing acute from maintenance treatment effects

Note. C = combined therapy. D = pharmacotherapy alone. P = psychotherapy alone. d = placebo only. p = attention control. Dp = pharmacotherapy plus attention control. Pd = psychotherapy plus placebo. cpd = attention control plus placebo. AMI = amitriptyline. TCA = tricyclic antidepressant. CMI = clomipramine. IMI = imipramine.

sion often treated in these studies (approximately half the subjects suffered from nonendogenous and/or situational depression). Yet, active drug was compared with placebo alone or placebo plus an attention control condition only three times. The absence of attention control conditions or attention control plus placebo conditions in 11 studies likewise leaves in question whether specific or nonspecific factors are at work with the addition of psychotherapy to drug management.

Also in question is whether either psychotherapy or drug has been provided in adequate doses or duration. For example, is the modal research format of a 12-week trial of an antidepressant medication followed by a taper off medication an adequate trial of drug therapy as it might be delivered optimally in clinical practice? Clinical wisdom might dictate a more prolonged period of drug treatment during the acute and continuation phases and a lower maintenance dose achieved by a more gradual taper that could be modified should signs of relapse occur. Does the once-a-week psychotherapy format of most studies represent an adequate "dose," or would twice-a-week psychotherapy be more effective (G. Klerman, M.D., personal communication)?

Another question that arises from this research is whether the investigators are capturing all the relevant aspects of therapeutic change attributable to the various treatment modalities. The most frequent outcome measures, the HRSD and the BDI (used in 12 and 10 of the 17 studies, respectively), may lack the necessary specificity to detect important areas of therapeutic effect. High, and often unbalanced, subject attrition (ranging from 25 to 50%) further compromises the interpretation of study results.

Major methodological issues that arise in reviewing this literature are twofold. First, there is great variability between studies on several dimensions. Most obvious is the fact that a number of different psychotherapies are used in combination with drug treatment. It is clearly less than optimal to lump together for the purpose of analysis studies using psychotherapies with such divergent theoretical underpinnings as cognitive-behavior therapy and interpersonal therapy. However, there are at present too few studies using any single therapeutic approach to draw robust conclusions. Variability of drug used was less of an issue, as 14 of 17 of the studies employed a tricyclic antidepressant only and 2 of the remaining 3 included a tricyclic antidepressant among two or more antidepressants used.

Comparing results across studies would have been facilitated also by a greater uniformity in the types and numbers of treatment cells in the comparisons that are made. For example, the characteristics of the attention control conditions showed little equivalence across studies.

The range spanned "nonscheduled treatment" (Weissman 1979), which consisted of telephone contact with a therapist whenever the subject felt the need, to half-hour "structured sessions" (Friedman 1975) for 7 of 12 weeks. As mentioned earlier, there was also relatively little overlap in the outcome measures used, with the exception of the HRSD and the BDI.

Variability also marked subject characteristics. Sample size ranged from 18 to 230; severity of depression, though defined almost uniformly by a HRSD score of greater than 14 of 17 and a BDI score of greater than 20, ranged from primarily "neurotic" (Covi et al. 1974; Friedman 1975) to predominantly severe (Hollon and Najavits 1988). Chronicity varied as well, from 6 months or less (Hollon and Najavits 1988) to 50 months (Hersen et al. 1984). There was also a great range in the methodological soundness of individual studies.

All of these problems in aggregating this literature, when added to the already mentioned inability to use metanalytic approaches, should encourage caution in interpreting results.

RESULTS

Having detailed the limitations in reviewing this literature, what conclusions can we extract from the studies, individually and as a whole, concerning the place of combined pharmacotherapy and psychotherapy in the treatment of depression? Does the coupling of drug and psychotherapy effect a greater overall reduction in depression and depression-related symptoms than does either component alone? Does it work more rapidly? Does it impact more effectively on specific patient subgroups or symptom domains? Does it enhance patient compliance?

To answer the question as to relative overall effectiveness, we tallied the outcomes for the individual studies as a function of both type of therapy employed and phase of treatment. In almost all instances, our reading of the results coincided with that of the authors. Results reflect mean response rates and universality, as differences between these two indices were not found on the whole. We did not discriminate between social, work, and other related measures and those of depressive symptomatology per se. We did not attempt to segregate studies according to type of drug used but instead lumped all drugs together, because most studies used a tricyclic antidepressant, most commonly imipramine or amitriptyline.

Turning first to a breakdown of study results by type of psychotherapy used (Table 1-7), note that we did not include in the grid a category in which combined therapy is less effective than component treatments. This is because in no study was there such a result. Only two studies described possible interference effects between pharmacotherapy and psychotherapy, and these were equivocal. In one (Bellack et al. 1981), data analysis on the first 72 of the final 120 patients sampled revealed that social skills training plus placebo resulted in a higher percentage of treatment responders compared with social skills training plus amitriptyline, amitriptyline alone, or dynamic psychotherapy plus placebo. However, when data on the full patient sample were evaluated, this finding was no longer apparent. In the second trial (Becker and Heimberg 1987), patients in the social skills training plus nortriptyline condition fared significantly less well than patients in all other conditions in only 1 of 13 symptom measures at midtreatment. Although the data suggesting negative interactions are at present unconvincing, the fact that both these studies used social skills training is worthy of note. Nonetheless, the conclusion that combination therapy is not less effective than pharmacotherapy or psychotherapy alone is perhaps the most robust finding we can report. This is an important result especially because it was once commonly taught that medication might interfere with the effects of psychotherapy and some psychopharmacologists have believed that psychotherapy might interfere with drug efficacy. Apparently, at the least, medication and psychotherapy do not get in each other's way.

Examining Table 1-7 further, it becomes clear that it is impossible to comment on the differential efficacy of combined treatment as a function of the five different psychotherapy disciplines employed. Unfortunately, at present, there are too few studies in each psychotherapy category to draw meaningful conclusions. We await the accumulation of more studies using each domain for the possible emergence of a particularly felicitous marriage of specific drugs and specific psychotherapies.

Table 1-7. Cell comparisons versus type of psychotherapy

	C > D	C = D	C > P	C = P
Psychoanalytic	0	1	3	1
Marital	0	1	0	1
Behavior	0	2	0	3
Interpersonal	1	1	1	1
Cognitive	3	1	3	5
Total	4	6	7	11

Note. C = combined therapy. D = pharmacotherapy alone.
P = psychotherapy alone.

If we sum all studies irrespective of the type of therapy used, we see that the combination approach outperformed drug treatment (i.e., drug alone and drug plus attention control conditions) in 4 of 10 instances, or 40% of the time. Combined therapy was found superior to psychotherapy (i.e., psychotherapy alone or with placebo) in 7 of 18 instances, or 39% of the time. Looked at another way, drug and psychotherapy given together were equivalent to drug alone 60% of the time and to psychotherapy alone 61% of the time.

It would seem that the evidence to date does not strongly support that combined therapy is necessary or desirable for all unipolar depressed outpatients, but that overall, it may be superior to individual treatments delivered alone. The suggestion of some advantage but the lack of overwhelming superiority for combined over single-modality approaches suggests that it may have a unique place in the treatment of some but not all patients. Who are these patients? What specific areas of advantage does combined therapy have over pharmacotherapy or psychotherapy alone in treating these patients?

Turning to individual study results, most authors initiate discussion of their data with an analysis of patient dropout patterns. It is indeed important to know whether patient attrition impacts on overall outcome and differs across groups. Most important, does the analysis of attrition patterns suggest trends in patient-treatment selection revealing differential suitability of treatment modalities by patient characteristics? As mentioned earlier, reported subject attrition rates run from 25 to 50%. With one-quarter to one-half of patients dropping out sometime in the course of treatment, it must be asked whether those who completed the protocol are representative of the original sample. Did completers differ from noncompleters as a whole on pretreatment variables such as demographic factors, severity of illness, etc.? Was differential cell dropout biasing the outcome? All but two authors reporting on attrition rates found no difference between study completers and noncompleters with respect to pretreatment variables (Beck et al. 1985; Covi and Lipman 1987; Friedman 1975; Hersen et al. 1984; Hollon and Najavits 1988; Murphy et al. 1984; Roth et al. 1982; Weissman et al. 1981). In one study (Blackburn et al. 1981), completers were found to be less depressed and less well educated than noncompleters. However, Hersen's group (Last et al. 1985) found completers to be more intelligent, more highly educated, and better adjusted socially than noncompleters. All but one of the authors found attrition to be nondifferential according to treatment condition (Beck et al. 1985; Blackburn et al. 1981; Covi and Lipman 1987; Friedman 1975; Hollon and Najavits 1988; Murphy et al. 1984; Roth et al. 1982). The aforementioned report from the Hersen study (Last et al. 1985) stated that endogenously depressed patients dropped out significantly less from the amitrip-tyline-alone condition than did nonendogenously depressed patients. When the two active drug-containing cells (social skills training plus amitriptyline and amitriptyline alone) were combined and compared with the remaining cells (social skills training plus placebo and short-term psychotherapy plus placebo), melancholic patients were found to have a higher completion rate in treatments including active drug. Another study suggests that combined therapy may result in higher patient retention than single-modality treatments: Murphy et al. (1984) discovered that, although there was no differential attrition by cell, collapsing cells into single- versus combined-modality treat-ment revealed a lower dropout rate for the latter.

A clue to the motivation behind patient attrition may be the data on patients' satisfaction with the treatment they receive. Weissman et al. (1981) found a higher rate of treatment refusal among patients randomized to psychotherapy than to drug therapy. Hollon and Najavits (1988) found this as a trend as well and pointed out a possible advantage for combined therapy over single-modality treatment in this context—i.e., that patients can refuse half of the therapy package and still stay in treatment. Similarly, Roth et al. (1982) noted that several patients undergoing combined therapy stated that they would have discontinued drug if it had not been for the psychotherapy component. In Hersen et al.'s study (1984), more severely depressed patients, especially those with melancholia, were relatively more dissatisfied with lack of early improvement in psychotherapy, whereas less depressed patients were relatively more intolerant of medication side effects. Wilson (1982) noted that over one-half of dropouts cited medication side effects as their reason for dropping out, whereas in another study, Friedman (1975) found side effects not to be a prominent reason given for attrition. Although most investigators found no statistically significant differences in attrition between treat-ment conditions, there remains the possibility, given the small sample sizes per cell, that a subtle self-selection process occurs during the course of treatment trials. It may be that patients who, for whatever reason, are more suited to their assigned treatment complete the trial, whereas those less well suited drop out, thereby making all com-parison conditions appear spuriously equivalent. Regardless of why patients fail to complete treatment in these trials, there is a large reservoir of patients who fall between the cracks. Combined therapy may aid overall treatment compliance, but it is by no means a fully satisfactory solution to this vexing problem.

Depression can be described along several dimensions: acute, chronic or intermittent, mild to severe, endogenous or nonendogenous, situational or nonsituational, etc. Do individual and combination treatments overlap in their effectiveness along each of these dimensions, or does each treatment format target depressive subtypes in a different manner? Unfortunately, the literature does not provide much data on differential response pattern according to depressive subtype. Five of the 17 studies we reviewed addressed this issue. Three of them (Beck et al. 1985; Blackburn et al. 1981; Roth et al. 1982) failed to find the presence or absence of endogenous features predictive of differential treatment response. However, Weissman et al. (1981) found endogenicity to be correlated with superior effectiveness of combined therapy relative to interpersonal therapy alone. In further separating endogenous patients into situational and nonsituational, the latter group showed an even stronger pattern of differential treatment response. Weissman et al. concluded that combination therapy may be most suited to the needs of the endogenously depressed patient, whereas single-modality therapy may be sufficient for nonendogenous patients.

Hollon's group (Garvey et al. 1985) looked at a number of depressive dimensions and discovered some interesting relationships. Along the dimension of severity, they found that less depressed patients fared better than did more severely depressed patients in the drug-alone conditions. More severely depressed patients responded better to combined therapy than to drug alone. Mild to moderately depressed patients did well in all therapy conditions. Presence of family history of depression augured better for the relative effectiveness of the combined condition over cognitive therapy alone. Family history of mania was associated with better response to combination therapy than to drug alone. Drug responders were more likely to be dexamethasone suppression test (DST) nonsuppressors than suppressors. DST status did not, however, predict differential response to cognitive therapy. Degree of cognitive dysfunction also did not predict differential treatment response.

Depressive suffering can be such that rapid onset of therapeutic effect is highly desirable. One of the assumptions behind the use of combined therapy in clinical practice is that two treatments may work faster than one. Do the study results support this assumption? Authors of two studies found combined therapy to produce earlier symptom reduction than comparative treatments (Blackburn et al. 1981; Roth et al. 1982). Three others found drug therapy to work more rapidly than psychotherapy, supporting the notion that the addition of drug to psychotherapy reduces the latency of therapeutic effect (Friedman 1975; Klerman et al. 1974; Weissman et al. 1981). In only one study

(Hollon and Najavits 1988), reporting on timing of effect, was no difference between treatments in this regard found. Although Hollon's group did not find combined treatment to work more rapidly than single-modality treatment, they did find another advantage for the combined approach. Although all active treatments resulted in significant symptom reduction in the 0- to 6-week phase of therapy, only combined treatment showed continued significant symptom reduction from 6 to 12 weeks. In sum, there is some evidence pointing to the fact that the addition of drug to psychotherapy can lead to an enhanced rapidity of symptomatic relief. Combined therapy may also result in therapeutic gains over a longer period. The evidence is not conclusive, however.

Pharmacotherapy and psychotherapy are so different in their nature and execution that they might well be presumed to impact on different symptom domains. If so, could these differences in effect work in a complementary way when the two therapies are combined? Again, no clear consensus emerges from the literature, but there are suggestive trends. Klerman et al. (1974) found that the interpersonal therapy component preferentially enhanced work and social functioning late in treatment. Marital therapy was found superior to drug treatment in restoring family role functioning, whereas drug treatment was more effective in reducing depressive symptoms (Friedman 1975). Weissman et al. (1981) confirmed Friedman's observations with interpersonal therapy and amitriptyline. Hersen et al. (1984) found social skills training to be associated with greater enhancement of interpersonal skills than was drug therapy. Covi and Lipman, in their more recent study (1987), noted differential reduction of phobic anxiety and somatization favoring combination therapy over psychotherapy alone. However, three other authors (Beck et al. 1985; Blackburn et al. 1981; Murphy et al. 1984) who looked at the question of differential treatment effects by symptom domain failed to distinguish between any active therapies.

In summary, there is some suggestion that if differential effects are indeed present, psychotherapy has stronger impact on social and role functioning, whereas drug therapy preferentially targets somatic symptoms of depression. Mainly however, pharmacotherapy and psychotherapy appear to overlap in their effects on depression and depression-related symptoms. Patients who improve tend to improve in a more global fashion regardless of the treatment delivered.

An important dimension to consider when evaluating the overall effectiveness of a treatment for depression is its durability. Because depression frequently presents in a recurring or chronic form, the longer-term continuation and maintenance treatment effects are of

similar importance to acute effects. Does the combination of pharmacotherapy and psychotherapy enhance the "immunity" to depressive relapse and/or recurrence conferred by either component
treatment delivered alone? The resolution of this question is confounded by a lack of clarity in the combination therapy literature as
to the period of risk for relapse versus recurrence and the potential
differential impact of various treatment conditions on this. However,
given this caveat, what does the literature tell us?

In a tally of overall outcome as a function of treatment phase (Table
1-8), there are 24 acute-phase, 6 continuation, 0 maintenance, and
12 follow-up treatment comparisons reported so far. The preponderance of combination therapy studies focus on the acute phase,
with fair attention given to follow-up. We are again reminded of the
paucity of continuation- and maintenance-phase trials, leaving us in
the dark as to the place of extended combination versus single-
modality treatment in bringing about more complete recovery in
partial responders to acute treatment and in preventing relapse and
recurrence. Nonetheless, a comparison of acute-phase results with
those at follow-up illustrates the relative immunizing effect of the
various treatment approaches against symptom reemergence. Although these studies are too few to be definite, the advantage of
combined psychotherapy and pharmacotherapy delivered in the acute
phase of depression over either treatment component alone appears
not to hold up over the long term, and the therapy component
appears to outdistance the drug component in this regard. Specifically, although Blackburn et al. (1981) found all treatment conditions
to be equivalent in mean amount of symptom reduction at 6-month
follow-up, they found a higher percentage of patients still in remission
in cognitive therapy with or without drug than in the drug-alone
condition. Weissman et al. (1981) noted enhanced social functioning
in patients who received interpersonal therapy with or without drug
treatment at 1-year follow-up. Murphy et al. (1984) found no sig-

Table 1-8. Cell comparisons versus phase of treatment

	C > D	C = D	C > P	C = P
Acute	4	6	5	9
Continuation	0	3	0	3
Maintenance	0	0	0	0
Follow-up	2	3	0	7

Note.   C = combined therapy. D = pharmacotherapy alone.
P = psychotherapy alone.

nificant difference in relapse rate by treatment cell, but when they applied the strict criterion for remission of a BDI score of less than 4, the relapse rate was significantly less for patients receiving cognitive therapy. Two other groups of investigators (Beck et al. 1985; Roth et al. 1982) found no superiority for the combination of drug and psychotherapy over the latter alone at 1-year follow-up. One important limitation applies to this set of conclusions. Most studies utilized a 12-week acute-phase trial of treatment with cessation of drug treatment at the end of that period. A 3-month drug-only trial may not reflect clinical practice. The one study that included a long-term drug therapy condition found that it was equivalent to short-term psychotherapy in preventing symptomatic failure (Hollon and Najavits 1988).

CONCLUSION

The question of the relative overall and specific advantage of combined treatment versus psychotherapy or medication alone is crucial. Depression has a high mortality and morbidity rate, and many patients are incomplete or nonresponders to one modality delivered alone. It would be very useful to know if, and for which patients, a combination approach will have the possible advantage of reduced dropout rates, increased spectrum of effect, or more profound impact.

Unfortunately, this is an especially difficult research question, not so much because it requires a particularly sophisticated design but because it is quite cumbersome to conduct. Large sample sizes are essential for two reasons: 1) there is little room at the top because the combination treatment is compared with already effective treatments and 2) many treatment cells are necessary to provide interpretable results. One design feature that perhaps should inform future studies is the choice of patient samples representing those who have already failed to respond to one treatment alone. This would increase the room for variance in improvement and address the question that is of perhaps greatest importance to the clinician concerning the use of combined treatment.

What conclusions can we draw from our interpretation of the available literature? The most obvious conclusion is that combined treatment appears to be at least as effective as psychotherapy or pharmacotherapy delivered alone. This is important in contradicting any accepted belief that psychotherapy would be rejected if a patient is on medication or vice versa. Even this conclusion must be moderated, however. Combined treatment is clearly more expensive and may have more side effects than a single-modality approach and

Table 1-9. Previous reviews of combination studies

Review study	No. of studies	Years included	No. of studies included in previous review	Type of analysis used by reviewer	Conclusion
Hollon and Beck 1978	4(31)[a]	1955–1977		Narrative	Cognitive is only therapy with specific effect on reducing depressive symptoms; need to look at cognitive therapy and drug; in general, C may broaden spectrum of response; only possible negative D/P interaction is therapy combined with placebo.
Weissman 1979	5(17)[a]	1974–1979	3	Narrative	C > D or P and is treatment of choice on average. C additive in that D and P work on different aspects of depressive syndrome. Negative interactions between P and D not found.
Conte et al. 1986	11	1974–1984	6	Modified metanalysis	70–85% of cell comparisons resulted in parity between C and other active treatment conditions, whereas remainder showed C to be superior.
Jarrett and Rush 1986	8	1974–1985	8	Narrative	Cognitive therapy and D may only exceed cognitive therapy alone in selected patients. Studies combining interpersonal therapy with D suggest that C > P or D alone for endogenous patients and may increase patient acceptance and compliance with treatment.

Hollon and Beck 1986	6[b]	1974–1985	6	Narrative	C > P or D alone, although findings are equivocal. There may be too little "room at the top" to detect much enhanced effect of C over P alone. Acute cognitive therapy seems more lasting in effect than D.
Weissman et al. 1987	12(2)[c]	1974–1987	10	Narrative	C still appears superior to P or D alone although not as robustly as earlier studies suggest.
Shea et al. 1988	12	1974–1986	12	Box score	Data do not provide strong support for superiority of C over D or P in reducing depressive symptoms. Small Ns limit conclusions.

Note. C = combined therapy. D = pharmacotherapy alone. P = psychotherapy alone.
[a]Number in parentheses indicates studies that either are inclusive of other diagnoses or do not have combination cells.
[b]Only studies employing cognitive therapy were included.
[c]Number in parentheses indicates studies that are in progress.

so must eventually justify increased cost and risk with greater likelihood of success.

There are suggestions in this literature that combined therapy is more effective than single-modality treatment and that the single modalities may have the kind of specific additive effects one would expect from them (i.e., medications preferentially improving somatic symptoms; psychotherapy improving cognitions or social maladjustment). There is also some suggestion that medications work more quickly but that psychotherapy is more durable—again an expected finding. We will, however, need many more studies before we can be confident that combined treatment is more effective or that the components have specific targets and/or durations of effect. The current literature certainly justifies such further research and also the current clinical practice of use of combined treatment particularly for the more difficult or nonresponding patient.

We have summarized in Table 1-9 the seven previous reviews that have been performed in this literature. It is of some interest that the ratio of reviews to actual studies is about 1:2.5, perhaps illustrating both the interest in the topic and the difficulty performing studies. Most of the reviews were narrative, although one other (Shea et al. 1988) used a box-score approach like ours, and Conte et al. (1986) attempted a modified metanalysis. The reviews are consistent in finding combined treatment to be at least equal to either treatment alone. More recent reviews (like ours) are somewhat less optimistic about the documentation of superior effect for combined treatment or of particular specific effects for the components. It is hoped that future reviews will have many additional studies and comparisons with the presentation of sufficient raw data to allow full-fledged metanalytic aggregation.

REFERENCES

Beck AT: Depression Inventory. Philadelphia, PA, Philadelphia Center for Cognitive Therapy, 1978

Beck AL, Hollon SD, Young JE, et al: Treatment of depression with cognitive therapy and amitriptyline. Arch Gen Psychiatry 42:142–148, 1985

Becker RE, Heimberg RG: Dysthymia: preliminary results of treatment with social skills training, crisis supportive psychotherapy, nortriptyline and placebo. Unpublished paper, 1987

Bellack AS, Hersen M, Himmelhoch J: Social skills training compared with pharmacotherapy in the treatment of unipolar depression. Am J Psychiatry 138:1562–1567, 1981

Bellack AS, Hersen M, Himmelhoch JM: A comparison of social skills training, pharmacotherapy, and psychotherapy for depression. Behav Res Ther 21:107–111, 1983

Beutler LE, Scogin F, Kirkish P, et al: Group cognitive therapy and alprazolam in the treatment of depression in older adults. J Consult Clin Psychol 55:550–556, 1987

Blackburn IM, Bishop S: Changes in cognition with pharmacotherapy and cognitive therapy. Br J Psychiatry 143:609–617, 1983

Blackburn IM, Bishop S, Glen AIM, et al: The efficacy of cognitive therapy in depression: a treatment trial using cognitive therapy and pharmacotherapy, each alone, and in combination. Br J Psychiatry 139:181–189, 1981

Blackburn IM, Evenson KM, Bishop S: A two-year naturalistic follow-up of depressed patients treated with cognitive therapy, pharmacotherapy and a combination of both. J Affective Disord 10:67–75, 1986

Cohen J: Statistical Power Analysis for the Behavioral Sciences. New York, Academic, 1969

Conte HR, Plutchik R, Wild KV, et al: Combined psychotherapy and pharmacotherapy for depression. Arch Gen Psychiatry 43:471–479, 1986

Covi L, Lipman RS: Cognitive behavioral group psychotherapy combined with imipramine in major depression. Psychopharmacol Bull 23:173–176, 1987

Covi L, Lipman RS, Derogatis LR, et al: Drugs and group psychotherapy in neurotic depression. Am J Psychiatry 131:191–198, 1974

Daneman EA: Imipramine in office management of depressive reactions. Diseases of the Nervous System 122:213–217, 1961

DiMascio A, Weissman MM, Prusoff BA, et al: Differential symptom reduction by drugs and psychotherapy in acute depression. Arch Gen Psychiatry 36:1450–1456, 1979

Evans MD, Hollon SD, DeRubeis RJ, et al: Accounting for relapse in a treatment outcome study of depression. Paper presented at the annual meeting of the Association for the Advancement of Behavior Therapy, November 16, 1985

Frank E, Kupfer DJ: Efficacy of combined imipramine and interpersonal psychotherapy. Psychopharmacol Bull 23:4–7, 1987

Friedman AS: Interaction of drug therapy with marital therapy in depressive patients. Arch Gen Psychiatry 32:619–637, 1975

Garvey MJ, Hollon SD, DeRubeis RJ, et al: Prediction of response to pharmacotherapy, cognitive therapy, and combined cognitive-pharmacotherapy, II: predicting response in the CPT project. Unpublished manuscript, University of Minnesota and the St. Paul-Ramsey Medical Center, Minneapolis–St. Paul, MN, 1985

Hamilton M: Development of a rating scale for primary depressive illness. British Journal of Social and Clinical Psychology 6:278–296, 1967

Hersen M, Bellack JM, Thase ME: Effects of social skill training, amitriptyline and psychotherapy in unipolar depressed women. Behavior Therapy 15:21–40, 1984

Hollon SD, Beck AT: Psychotherapy and drug therapy: comparison and combinations, in Handbook of Psychotherapy and Behavior Change: An Empirical Analysis, 2nd Edition. Edited by Garfield SL, Bergin AE. New York, John Wiley, 1978, pp 437–490

Hollon SD, Beck AT: Cognitive and cognitive-behavioral therapies, in Handbook of Psychotherapy and Behavior Change, 3rd Edition. Edited by Garfield SL, Bergin AE. New York, John Wiley, 1986, pp 443–482

Hollon SD, DeRubeis RJ: Placebo-psychotherapy combinations: inappropriate representations of psychotherapy in drug-psychotherapy comparative trials. Psychol Bull 90:467–477, 1981

Hollon SD, Najavits L: Review of empirical studies on cognitive therapy, in American Psychiatric Press Review of Psychiatry, Vol 7. Edited by Frances AJ, Hales RE. Washington, DC, American Psychiatric Press, 1988, pp 643–666

Jarrett RB, Rush AJ: Psychotherapeutic approaches for depression, in Psychiatry, Vol 1. Edited by Cavener JO. New York, Basic Books, 1986

Klerman GL, DiMascio A, Weissman MM, et al: Treatment of depression by drugs and psychotherapy. Am J Psychiatry 131:186–191, 1974

Last CG, Thase ME, Hersen M, et al: Patterns of attrition for psychosocial and pharmacological treatments of depression. J Clin Psychiatry 46:361–366, 1985

Murphy GE, Simmons AD, Wetzel RD, et al: Cognitive therapy and pharmacotherapy. Arch Gen Psychiatry 41:33–41, 1984

Paykel ES, DiMascio A, Haskell D, et al: Effects of maintenance amitriptyline and psychotherapy on symptoms of depression. Psychol Med 5:67–77, 1975

Prusoff BA, Weissman MM, Klerman GL, et al: Research Diagnostic Criteria subtypes of depression. Arch Gen Psychiatry 37:796–801, 1980

Roth D, Bielski R, Jones M, et al: A comparison of self control therapy and antidepressant medication in the treatment of depression. Behavior Therapy 13:133–144, 1982

Rothblum ED, Sholomskas AJ, Berry C, et al: Issues in clinical trials with the depressed elderly. Br J Psychiatry 30:695–699, 1982

Rounsaville BJ, Klerman GL, Weissman MM: Do psychotherapy and pharmacotherapy for depression conflict? Empirical evidence from a clinical trial. Arch Gen Psychiatry 38:24–29, 1981

Rush AJ, Watkins JT: Group versus individual cognitive therapy: a pilot study. Cognitive Therapy Research 5:95–103, 1981

Shea MT, Elkin I, Hirschfeld RMA: Psychotherapeutic treatment of depression, in American Psychiatric Press Review of Psychiatry, Vol 7. Edited by Frances AJ, Hales RE. Washington, DC, American Psychiatric Press, 1988, pp 235–255

Simons AD, Murphy GE, Levine JL, et al: Cognitive therapy and pharmacotherapy for depression. Arch Gen Psychiatry 43:43–48, 1986

Teasdale JD, Fennell MJV, Hibbert GA, et al: Cognitive therapy for major depressive disorder in primary care. Br J Psychiatry 144:400–406, 1984

Weissman MM: The psychological treatment of depression. Arch Gen Psychiatry 36:1261–1269, 1979

Weissman MM, Klerman GL, Paykel ES, et al: Treatment effects on the social adjustment of depressed patients. Arch Gen Psychiatry 30:771–778, 1974

Weissman MM, Prusoff BA, DiMascio A, et al: The efficacy of drugs and psychotherapy in the treatment of acute depressive episodes. Am J Psychiatry 136:555–558, 1979

Weissman MM, Klerman GL, Prusoff BA, et al: Depressed outpatients: one year after treatment with drugs and/or interpersonal psychotherapy. Arch Gen Psychiatry 38:51–55, 1981

Weissman MM, Jarrett RB, Rush AJ: Psychotherapy and its relevance to the pharmacotherapy of major depression: a decade later (1976–1985), in Psychopharmacology: The Third Generation of Progress. Edited by Meltzer H, Coyle JT, Kopin IJ, et al. New York, Raven, 1987

Wilson PH: Combined pharmacological and behavioral treatment of depression. Behav Res Ther 20:173–184, 1982

Chapter 2

Combined Cognitive Therapy and Pharmacotherapy in the Treatment of Depression

Steven D. Hollon, Ph.D.
Robert J. DeRubeis, Ph.D.
Mark D. Evans, Ph.D.

Chapter 2

Combined Cognitive Therapy and Pharmacotherapy in the Treatment of Depression

Therapists interested in the treatment of depression frequently consider combining two distinct forms of treatment, pharmacotherapy and psychotherapy. The literature has long supported the efficacy of the antidepressant medications in the treatment of depression, particularly the tricyclics (Klein and Davis 1967; Morris and Beck 1974). Initial attempts to document the efficacy of the psychotherapies were less than wholly supportive. Although approaches such as supportive group therapy (Covi et al. 1974), marital therapy (Friedman 1975), and interpersonal counseling (Klerman et al. 1974) were shown to affect problem areas other than depression, those interventions were each less effective than pharmacotherapy alone, and none of them enhanced efficacy when added to medications (Hollon and Beck 1978; Uhlenhuth et al. 1969).

This picture has changed over the last decade with respect to the psychosocial interventions. Although the tricyclic antidepressants remain the standard treatment for nonpsychotic, nonbipolar-depressed outpatients, several types of psychosocial interventions have been shown to be effective, including cognitive therapy (Beck et al. 1985; Blackburn et al. 1981; Covi and Lipman 1987; Elkin et al. 1986; Murphy et al. 1984; Rush et al. 1977; Teasdale et al. 1984),

Preparation of this chapter was supported by Grant MH-33209 from the National Institute of Mental Health. This chapter was read in part before the 141st annual meeting of the American Psychiatric Association, Montreal, 12 May 1988. We thank Vicente B. Tuason, M.D., Michael J. Garvey, M.D., William M. Grove, Ph.D., Marlin J. Wiemer, Ph.D., and Joan M. Piasecki, B.A., who were co-investigators on the comparative treatment outcome study described in this chapter.

interpersonal psychotherapy (Elkin et al. 1986; Weissman et al. 1979), and various other approaches (Bellack et al. 1981; McLean and Hakstian 1979; Roth et al. 1982).

Given that both psychosocial and pharmacological treatments are effective in the treatment of at least some depressions, it is reasonable that therapists and researchers have begun combining the two. In fact, although no good survey of present clinical practice currently exists, it is generally assumed that pragmatic combinations of drugs and psychosocial interventions are widely used in the larger treatment community. Theoretically based speculations regarding the potential negative consequences of combining the two modalities used to be commonly accepted (see Klerman 1986, for a review), but have not been supported by more recent controlled clinical trials (see, for example, Rounsaville et al. 1981). Nonetheless, there is a paucity of controlled data on the comparative efficacy of combined treatments relative to the two single modalities.

In this chapter, we describe a recent controlled empirical trial contrasting tricyclic pharmacotherapy versus cognitive therapy, each alone and in combination, in the treatment of depression. We evaluated the two single modalities vis-à-vis the combination with respect to several aspects of outcome (Hollon 1981). These included the reduction of acute symptomatology for the average treated patient (*magnitude*), the number of patients within a given modality who evidenced an adequate response (*universality*), and the extent to which treatment gains were maintained after treatment cessation (*stability*). We were further interested in identifying any potential indicators of differential response or relapse (*prescriptive indices*), because the identification of such markers can facilitate matching individual patients to their optimal treatment. In addition, we were concerned with the extent to which the respective treatments were free from attrition (*acceptability*), as well as the extent to which the respective treatments were free from undesirable complications (*safety*). Finally, we sought to determine which aspects of the complex treatment packages used truly accounted for the changes observed, both with respect to the active ingredients in each modality (*components*) and the client processes that mediated those interventions' impacts (*mechanisms*).

PRIOR RESEARCH INVOLVING COGNITIVE THERAPY

In 1977, Rush et al. published a controlled trial in which cognitive therapy was found to be superior to imipramine tricyclic pharmacotherapy. In that 12-week-long comparison, nonpsychotic, nonbipolar-depressed outpatients responded better to cognitive therapy than to imipramine pharmacotherapy plus supportive clinical management. Attrition rates were also lower in the cognitive therapy treatment condition. Finally, patients treated with cognitive therapy evidenced a nonsignificantly lower rate of relapse across a 1-year follow-up (Kovacs et al. 1981). Although this study created considerable interest in cognitive therapy in the literature, it created considerable controversy as well. There were several features of the Rush et al. design that reduced confidence in the findings. First, the study was conducted at the center at which cognitive therapy was developed. Even with the best of intentions, such a situation is particularly conducive to the operation of subtle biasing factors favoring the cognitive modality. Second, medication plasma levels were not checked, leaving open the possibility that noncompliance or nonabsorption might have undercut the efficacy of pharmacotherapy (Glassman et al. 1977; Gram et al. 1976). Third, and most critical, patients in the original trial were tapered from medications starting in week 10 of the 12-week protocol. The rationale for this procedure was a desire to have all patients be done with treatment by the end of week 12. Because it takes anywhere from several days to 2 weeks to eliminate all traces of tricyclic medication from the bloodstream, it seemed reasonable at the time to step pharmacotherapy-treated patients off of medications before the scheduled end of protocol treatment.

In retrospect, we think that Rush et al. (1977) confounded response to active treatment with relapse following treatment cessation. As shown in Figure 2-1, differences between cognitive therapy and tricyclic pharmacotherapy became particularly pronounced after medication withdrawal was begun in week 10 (the graph for the cognitively treated condition is extended through week 14, but all active treatment ceased in week 12). Several of the patients withdrawn from medications evidenced a return of depressive symptomatology during this period. This renewed symptomatology raised mean depression scores for the pharmacotherapy condition at the posttreatment evaluation, but such instances were not counted as relapses in the subsequent follow-up report because they occurred before the "end of treatment" (Kovacs et al. 1981).

In a subsequent study at this same center, Beck et al. (1985) found no differences between cognitive therapy alone and combined cognitive therapy–pharmacotherapy for depressed outpatients. Although the combined condition did not outperform cognitive therapy alone, it is not clear in retrospect that dosage levels of the tricyclic used, a maximum of 150 mg of amitriptyline per day, were fully clinically representative. In other combinatorial trials, combined cognitive therapy–pharmacotherapy has sometimes been superior to one or both of the single modalities (Blackburn et al. 1981; Teasdale et al. 1984) and at other times only equivalent (Murphy et al. 1984), but never inferior to either single modality.

COGNITIVE –PHARMACOTHERAPY PROJECT (CPT)

Starting in the late 1970s, our group began a major psychotherapy-pharmacotherapy project designed to evaluate the various dimensions of comparative and combinatorial efficacy just described. The project, referred to as the Cognitive-Pharmacotherapy Project (CPT), was conceived as a replication and extension of the earlier Rush et al. (1977) trial. Our goal was to provide an unbiased comparison between cognitive therapy and tricyclic pharmacotherapy, each alone and in combination, that was both rigorously controlled and fully representative of current clinical practice. The project was conducted concurrently in two settings, the St. Paul–Ramsey Medical Center, which has a long history of participation in nationally funded pharmacotherapy trials (Ling et al. 1984; Prien et al. 1984), and the Ramsey County Adult Mental Health Center, a community mental health center known in the region for its attention to the delivery of psychosocial treatment. Patients were drawn from people requesting treatment for depression at either setting. This not only ensured that the samples treated were clinically representative, it also guaranteed that the sample would consist of people seeking or expecting a variety

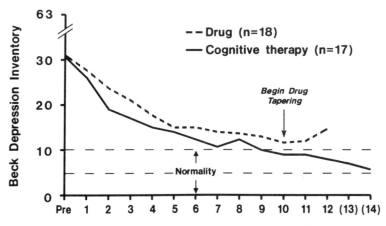

Figure 2-1. Outcome in Rush et al. (1977) study: weekly scores by group.

of forms of treatment. Similarly, the study therapists were drawn from the existing treatment staffs already in place in the two facilities, again serving to heighten clinical realism and balance potential biases across the two treatment modalities.

As described in an as yet unpublished manuscript by Hollon et al., the sample consisted of 107 primary, nonbipolar, nonpsychotic depressed outpatients. Potential patients were screened by a project evaluator on a modified version of the Schedule for Affective Disorders and Schizophrenia—Lifetime Version (SADS-L; Endicott and Spitzer 1978; Spitzer and Endicott 1979). Inclusion criteria included 1) major depressive disorder according to Research Diagnostic Criteria (RDC; Spitzer et al. 1978; Spitzer et al. 1979), 2) a score of 20 or above on the self-report Beck Depression Inventory (BDI; Beck et al. 1961), and 3) a score of 14 or above on the 17-item version of the clinician-rated Hamilton Rating Scale for Depression (HRSD; Hamilton 1960). Exclusion criteria included 1) past or current RDC diagnosis of schizophrenia, bipolar I affective disorder, organic brain syndrome, antisocial personality, panic disorder, or generalized anxiety disorder; 2) RDC diagnosis of alcoholism or drug abuse disorder within the last year; 3) hallucinations, delusions, or stupor; 4) suicide risk necessitating immediate hospitalization; 5) medical history or current laboratory tests contraindicating tricyclic pharmacotherapy; 6) recent (within 3 months) history of nonresponse to an adequate trial of imipramine (defined as 150 mg/day for at least 2 weeks); or 7) an IQ below 80. Patients were not excluded who met RDC criteria for minor depressive disorder or depressive, labile, or cyclothymic personality, so long as they also currently met criteria for major depression. This meant that the sample was heterogeneous with respect to the presence of "double depression." Similarly, the sample was heterogeneous with respect to personality disorder (other than antisocial personality), and both endogenous and nonendogenous subtypes of depression were represented.

Patients meeting all criteria and agreeing to participation were randomly assigned to treatment. Patients assigned to cognitive therapy received a maximum of twenty 50-minute sessions over a 12-week period. Cognitive therapy was conducted in accordance with the manual developed by Beck et al. (1979). The four cognitive therapists were all experienced psychotherapists with at least 8 years of clinical experience. All therapists treated several patients under project supervision before working with study patients. Ongoing supervision was provided in twice-weekly sessions throughout the bulk of the project.

Patients assigned to pharmacotherapy were seen once weekly, with the beginning session typically lasting about 50 minutes and subsequent sessions typically lasting about 20–30 minutes. Treatment was focused on 1) pharmacotherapy management, which involved educating patients about medications, adjusting dosage and dosage schedules, and inquiring about and dealing with side effects; and 2) clinical management, which involved a review of the patient's functioning in major life spheres, supportive counseling, and advice giving. All five project pharmacotherapists were experienced research psychiatrists who had taken part in previous controlled research trials. The pharmacotherapists met periodically under the supervision of the project medical director, Vicente B. Tuason, M.D., to review adherence to the treatment protocol.

The medication used in the study was imipramine hydrochloride, provided in flexible daily dosages, incrementing to 200–300 mg per day by week 3. Blood plasma levels were available to the pharmacotherapists, and medication dosage levels were raised above 300 mg per day in instances in which clinical response was not adequate and there was no risk of toxicity.

Patients assigned to combined cognitive therapy–pharmacotherapy received both modalities as described above. Each combined-condition patient worked with both a cognitive therapist and a pharmacotherapist. There were no differences in the number of cognitive therapy sessions between cognitive therapy alone versus combined cognitive therapy–pharmacotherapy (15.4 versus 14.4), the number of pharmacotherapy sessions (8.9 versus 8.8), or maximum drug dosage levels (239 versus 225 mg per day) between pharmacotherapy alone and combined cognitive therapy–pharmacotherapy. Past combinatorial trials have sometimes not equated the degree or amount of each respective component in the combined condition to the single modalities, a practice that would produce a conservative estimate of the efficacy of the combined treatment (Hollon and Beck 1978).

Acceptability

Sixty-four of the 107 patients screened into the trial completed the full 12-week treatment protocol. Five patients failed to begin treatment after randomization (3 in the cognitive therapy–alone condition), and another 38 patients dropped out of treatment after it was begun. Although attrition rates were high, ranging from 44% in the pharmacotherapy-only condition to 36% each in cognitive therapy alone and combined cognitive therapy–pharmacotherapy, they did not differ significantly across the treatment conditions. This indicates an absence of differential acceptability as a function of treatment modality. It may well be that the differential attrition rate noted in the original Rush et al. (1977) trial was a consequence of the expectation of receiving cognitive therapy on the part of patients seeking treatment at that facility. It should also be noted that although the attrition rates observed in the CPT study were uniformly high, they were not so high as the 50% attrition rate cited by Garfield (1978) for the typical community mental health center outpatient such as was treated in this project.

At the same time, there was an indication, albeit nonsignificant, that patients dropping out of combined treatment early in the trial (before completing more than 3 weeks) were more severely depressed than comparable early dropouts in the other conditions. Although this attrition came too early in the trial to represent an instance of treatment failure, it could well have biased subsequent comparisons in favor of the combined modalities. This is a point to which we will return in our discussion of acute response.

Response to Acute Treatment (Magnitude)

Figure 2-2 presents the group means for all patients completing

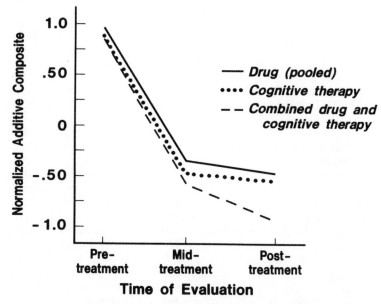

Figure 2-2. Change in depression on composite (Beck Depression Inventory, Hamilton Rating Scale for Depression, Raskin Depression Scale, and Minnesota Multiphasic Personality Inventory Self-report Scale 2 – depression).

treatment in the three treatment conditions (the two pharmacotherapy-only conditions are pooled, because treatment in those conditions was identical during the acute treatment phase). The depression composite depicted represents an unweighted additive composite across four measures of syndrome depression. The self-report BDI and clinician-rated HRSD have already been described. The other two measures were the self-report scale 2 (depression) of the Minnesota Multiphasic Personality Inventory (MMPI-D; Hathaway and McKinley 1951) and the clinician-rated Raskin Depression Scale (RDS; Raskin et al. 1970). Both clinician-rated scales were rated by independent clinicians blind to treatment condition.

Our rationale for combining the four syndrome depression measures was as follows. Because each is a widely used but fallible measure of syndrome depression, an additive composite based on the four should provide a psychometrically more satisfying index of the underlying construct of interest than any single measure (Horowitz et al. 1979). Further, the different measures emphasize different components of the larger syndrome (e.g., the BDI samples cognitive components more adequately than does the HRSD, whereas the HRSD samples vegetative components more adequately than does the BDI). By incorporating different measures of syndrome depression in the larger additive composite, we think we not only improved the properties of our measure psychometrically, but also substantively improved content coverage. Finally, by adopting the additive composite as our primary measure of syndrome depression, we were able to reduce the number of analyses experiment-wise, reducing the risk of finding significant differences simply on the basis of chance.

The unweighted additive composite was constructed by first normalizing each syndrome measure across the three assessment points: intake, midtreatment (6 weeks), and posttreatment (12 weeks). Scores across the four individual measures were then averaged for each patient at each assessment point. This averaging procedure had the additional advantage of handling missing data on any given measure without requiring the deletion of the particular case, a more satisfying procedure than the casewise deletion that would have occurred under the more conventional univariate or multivariate analysis of variance strategies. The resultant composite had a mean of 0 and a standard deviation of 1 across all three assessment points, with elevations at intake in the .90 range and subsequent midtreatment and posttreatment means in the −.45 and − .60 ranges, respectively.

As can be seen in Figure 2-2, all three groups evidenced comparable elevations on syndrome depression at intake (a composite score of .92 at intake corresponds to a BDI score of 30.6, a MMPI-D T-score of

83.4, a HRSD score of 24.1, and a RDS score of 10.5). These values are quite comparable to those evidenced in prior comparative trials using outpatient samples (e.g., Beck et al. 1985; Blackburn et al. 1981; Murphy et al. 1984; Rush et al. 1977). All three cells evidenced marked change over time, with the greatest change occurring between intake and midtreatment. Over 90% of the observed change in syndrome depression occurred over the first 6 weeks of treatment. There were no differences between the three conditions at midtreatment; all three conditions evidenced significant change from intake to midtreatment, but none evidenced either more rapid change or greater total change by the midtreatment evaluation. Only the combined condition continued to evidence significant change between the midtreatment and posttreatment evaluations. At posttreatment, combined treatment evidenced a nonsignificant trend relative to pharmacotherapy alone and a comparably sized advantage relative to cognitive therapy alone that fell just short of being a trend due to the smaller sample size. Effect sizes, calculated as the ratio of the differences between the means divided by the standard deviation, were moderate for both comparisons, equal to .66 and .58, respectively (Cohen 1969). This pattern was essentially replicated across the four univariate measures, with differences on the MMPI-D fully significant and only the BDI failing to evidence at least a nonsignificant trend favoring the combined condition over the single modalities.

These findings were essentially replicated when eventual dropouts who completed more than 3 weeks of treatment were included via end-point analysis. However, differences diminished somewhat (effect size = .37 and .34, respectively) when all patients initially assigned were included and no longer indicated even nonsignificant trends. Thus, as previously indicated, the nonsignificant tendency for more severely depressed patients to drop out of combined treatment before receiving an adequate exposure may have biased the comparison somewhat in favor of that combination. At the same time, differential effect sizes remained at least small to moderate, suggesting that the nonsignificant advantages evident among the completers only were not wholly produced by differential early attrition. Although differences of such a magnitude were not likely to be detected given the relatively small samples involved, they are not inconsequential and may well represent a modest, but important, advantage for the combination if replicated in subsequent studies with larger samples.

These findings suggest that combined cognitive therapy–pharmacotherapy may ultimately prove more effective than either single modality. The magnitude of the differences between the respective conditions was not great, but it was fairly robust across multiple measures. Combined treatment has not always proven superior to either single modality in other relevant studies, but it has typically produced at least some such indications. For example, Blackburn et al. (1981) found combined treatment to be superior to pharmacotherapy in both a general practice and a psychiatric outpatient sample and superior to cognitive therapy in the latter. The combined condition in the Murphy et al. (1984) trial evidenced some indication of greater rates of response relative to the single modalities, but these differences did not reach conventional levels of significance. In at least one other trial (Beck et al. 1985), the adequacy of the execution of the pharmacological component of the combined condition has been called into question. Given this pattern of findings, it may be that combined treatment will ultimately prove to be superior to either single modality in terms of reducing acute symptomatology.

Universality

Group data can be misleading with regard to outcome for individual patients (Jacobson et al. 1984). Although the "average" completer in each single modality ended treatment not more than a standard deviation above the mean for nondepressive patients, and the "average" patient in the combined condition approached the mean for nondepressive patients, such group means can mask considerable individual variability in response. When we classified patients into full response (posttreatment BDI scores ≤9), partial response (BDI scores between 10 and 15), and nonresponse (BDI scores ≥16), following conventions established by Rush et al. (1977) and Murphy et al. (1984), we found no differences between the three conditions. Seventy-five percent of the patients treated in either single modality evidenced full or partial response, with an increment to 88% in the combined modality. An examination of the pattern of individual results was most consistent with the hypothesis that combined treatment increased the number of patients who showed a clinical response, not the average response of the typical patient in the combined modality. If true, this would suggest that combined treatment is not superior for everyone, but rather that patients unlikely to respond to one or the other single modality are more likely to receive something they will respond to in the combination.

Safety

Three patients made suicide attempts during the course of the project; two died as a result. All attempts apparently involved study medications. Two of the patients making attempts (including one of the fatalities) had been assigned to pharmacotherapy alone, whereas the third patient attempting suicide (and the second fatality) was in the combined treatment condition. Two other patients were withdrawn from pharmacotherapy alone and hospitalized due to symptomatic worsening or acute suicidal crisis, and three other patients were withdrawn from the same condition due to severe medication reactions. Finally, one patient was withdrawn from cognitive therapy after exhibiting a manic episode of psychotic proportions in the 6th week of treatment. Although such instances were too few to warrant statistical analysis, eight of the nine patients exhibiting serious consequences associated with treatment were receiving pharmacotherapy— seven in pharmacotherapy alone and one in combined cognitive therapy–pharmacotherapy. Whether these patterns will be maintained in subsequent studies remains to be seen, but the possibility exists that differential safety indices will favor the psychosocial therapy–only condition.

Prediction of Differential Responses

We attempted to identify both prognostic and prescriptive indicators by casting a series of general linear models treating pretreatment depression (as indexed by the additive composite) as the covariate and posttreatment depression (as indexed by that same composite) as the dependent variable. Potential predictors included various demographic, history of illness, family history, depressive subtype, personality, biological, and cognitive indicators. This initial battery was first subjected to a series of factor analyses to reduce the number of potential predictors. A total of 23 univariate indices and multivariate factors were entered as independent variables in the individual equations.

As reported in an as yet unpublished manuscript by Garvey et al., there were few indicators of differential response. Patients who were married and/or employed at the beginning of the trial generally did better in treatment than did patients who were not, and this relationship held across all three treatment conditions. Patients with higher levels of initial symptomatology did better in combined treatment than in pharmacotherapy alone. Another way of interpreting this finding is to say that patients with only moderate or lower symptomatology did equally well in any of the treatment conditions. Severity of initial symptomatology also predicted response within the pharmacotherapy-alone condition, with less depressed patients doing better in pharmacotherapy alone than more depressed patients. Patients with family histories of depression did less well in cognitive therapy alone than they did in combined treatment. Patients with a positive family history of mania did significantly less well in pharmacotherapy alone than they did in either cognitive therapy or combined treatment.

Perhaps our most interesting findings with respect to differential prescription came from the biological domain. We had assessed both urinary 3-methoxy-4-hydroxyphenethyleneglycol (MHPG; based on two consecutive 24-hour urinary collections, corrected for creatine levels) and cortisol dysregulation, as indicated by the dexamethasone suppression test (DST; Carroll et al. 1981), as part of our initial screening battery. Female patients evidenced a nonsignificant tendency to differ in their response to pharmacotherapy versus combined treatment as a function of initial MHPG status. The bulk of the interaction was contributed by female patients high on pretreatment MHPG doing better in combined treatment than in pharmacotherapy alone (Figure 2-3). These same patients did worse in imipramine pharmacotherapy than did female patients evidencing lower MHPG levels at pretreatment. This latter finding is quite consistent with the existing literature (Bielski and Friedel 1976), but may be specific to the type of tricyclic used in the study.

DST nonsuppressors did significantly better than DST suppressors when patients receiving any medications (either alone or in combina-

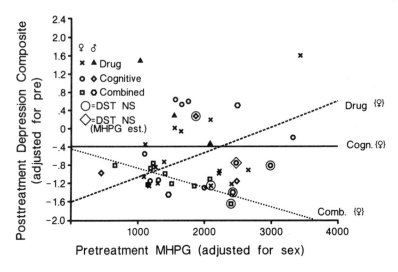

Figure 2-3.   Residualized posttreatment depression as a function of pre-treatment 3-methoxy-4-hydroxyphenethyleneglycol (MHPG; adjusted for sex). DST NS = dexamethasone suppression test nonsuppressors.

tion with cognitive therapy) were pooled (Figure 2-4). No such effect was evident within the cognitive therapy–alone condition. DST non-suppressors evidenced a nonsignificant trend for superior response to any modality that included pharmacotherapy relative to cognitive therapy alone. Because the DST nonsuppressors generally exhibited elevated pretreatment MHPG levels, this pattern of findings, in combination with the MHPG findings, suggests an interesting inter-action. In brief, it appears that DST status may moderate the MHPG-by-treatment trend previously described, with high scorers on MHPG doing worse in pharmacotherapy than in cognitive therapy alone or combined treatment unless they are also DST nonsuppressors. Elevated MHPG levels may well reflect an effort to compensate for a dysfunction in neurotransmitter systems other than norepinephrine, for example, serotonin or acetylcholine. Although imipramine is largely noradrenergic in its mechanism of action, it is not wholly so. MHPG elevations may prove to be multiply determined, with DST nonsuppression serving as a marker for those high-MHPG patients who are likely to be imipramine responsive.

This brings us to an important point regarding psychotherapy-

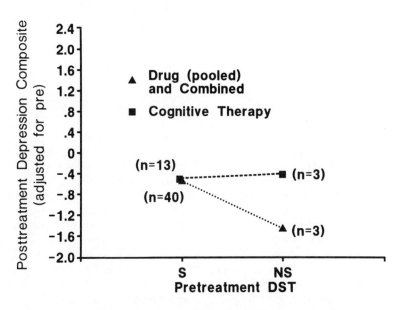

Figure 2-4. Residualized posttreatment depression as a function of pre-treatment dexamethasone suppression test (DST). S = sup-pressors. NS = nonsuppressors.

pharmacotherapy combinations: the relative efficacies of the specific combination may well prove to be a function of the specific types of single modalities included, not general characteristics of all possible combinations. Had we selected a tricyclic other than imipramine (e.g., one with a more targeted or different mechanism of action), we might have discovered a different pattern of differential response within our respective modalities and, possibly, a different pattern of overall response to the combination relative to the single modalities. Other studies have used different tricyclics. For example, Murphy et al. (1984) used nortriptyline and found no differences between either single modality and combined treatment, although, as noted earlier, visible differences favoring the combination were apparent, but not significant. Nortriptyline is presumed to be more purely serotonergic in its mechanism of action than is imipramine; it is possible that the lesser differences between pharmacotherapy alone and combined treatment reported in the Murphy et al. trial reflected a better response by the high-MHPG patients who were DST suppressors than was observed in the CPT project. Similarly, RDC endogenicity was not predictive of differential response in our CPT project, nor in any other trial involving cognitive therapy–pharmacotherapy comparisons or combinations in which it was examined (Blackburn et al. 1981; Kovacs et al. 1981; Simons et al. 1985). It was predictive of differential response in a recent trial contrasting interpersonal psychotherapy with amitriptyline, each alone and in combination (Prusoff et al. 1980). In that study, patients evidencing an endogenous subtype responded better to either pharmacotherapy alone or combined interpersonal psychotherapy–pharmacotherapy than they did to interpersonal psychotherapy alone, and patients evidencing a nonendogenous pattern responded better to either interpersonal psychotherapy alone or combined interpersonal psychotherapy–pharmacotherapy than they did to pharmacotherapy alone.

It remains quite possible that specific combinations of particular psychotherapies and pharmacologic agents will evidence differential patterns of response among particular subpopulations within the larger category of the nonpsychotic, nonbipolar depressive disorders. At this time, the combinatorial literature has not approached this issue in the kind of coordinated fashion that would permit an empirical answer to emerge (i.e., by varying the types of specific agents included in the respective trials in a systematic way). We think this is an important direction for future combinatorial research. At this time, there is little evidence for different absolute efficacies across the respective specific interventions within either single modality domain, with some indication that combinations across the two modality domains may at times, but not invariably, enhance overall efficacy. Whether specific combinations can be selected that enhance overall efficacy via matching the most effective intervention to the needs of the specific patient remains an intriguing line of inquiry (Paul 1967).

Before leaving the general issue of differential prediction, we want to comment on several of the variables that did not predict differential response, either within the specific modalities (prognostically) or across the different modalities (prescriptively). First, although we did assess general intelligence, socioeconomic status, and level of education, we found no relation between any of these variables and subsequent response. They did, independently and in combination, predict attrition across all of the treatment conditions. Less intelligent, lower socioeconomic status, less educated patients were more likely to drop out from any of the conditions than were patients evidencing higher levels of these three predictors, but they did not evidence differential attrition, nor did they evidence differential clinical response. It has long been assumed that such indicators should predict differentially poorer response for cognitive therapy, which is often presumed to require considerable intellectual capacity on the part of the patient to be effective. This assumption has never been borne out empirically in any trial in which it has been explored (e.g., Blackburn et al. 1981; Rush et al. 1978; Simons et al. 1985). Similarly, we found no evidence that variation in the degree of cognitive dysfunction at intake was at all predictive of subsequent clinical response. Again, this is generally consistent with prior research. To date, the only variable from the cognitive-personality domain that has been found to be a predictor of differential response to cognitive therapy versus pharmacotherapy has been "learned resourcefulness," a presumed indicator of readiness to exercise personal control over one's own psychological and behavioral processes (Rosenbaum 1980). Simons et al. (1985) reported that patients high on learned resourcefulness did significantly better in either cognitive therapy alone or combined cognitive therapy–pharmacotherapy than they did in pharmacotherapy alone, whereas patients low on this variable showed the opposite trend. Whether this relation will replicate across subsequent studies remains to be determined. For now, it remains the only suggestion of any differential prescriptive index deriving from the cognitive-personality domain.

Relapse After Treatment Cessation

We turn now to what we consider to be the most exciting finding emerging from the combined cognitive therapy–pharmacotherapy literature—the differential prevention of subsequent symptomatic relapse after successful treatment. Depression has long been recognized as being not only self-limiting, but also episodic (Beck 1967; Zis and Goodwin 1979). This means that although the typical depressed patient can be expected to recover from any given episode even in the absence of effective treatment, that same patient is at considerable risk of experiencing subsequent episodes at some future time. Although empirical data derived from naturalistic longitudinal studies are sparse and variability across individuals is great, it has been estimated that the typical episode will last about 6–9 months in outpatients and about 9–12 months in inpatients (Beck 1967). The average intermorbid interval between episodes appears to be about 3 years, with risk declining somewhat over time (Beck 1967; Lavori et al. 1984). Given the propensity for spontaneous remission in any given episode, but elevated risk for subsequent episodes, a strong case can be made that the reduction of future risk is as important as the successful treatment of the current episode.

It is in this regard that advocates of psychosocial interventions have long made the strongest claims. Few proponents of antidepressant pharmacotherapy have ever suggested that effective treatment reduced risk for subsequent symptomatology after the cessation of treatment. Although continuation and maintenance strategies do appear to prevent the emergence of subsequent episodes in both nonbipolar and bipolar types (Klerman 1978; Prien and Caffey 1977), it remains controversial whether that effect represents an instance of true prophylaxis as opposed to ongoing symptom suppression. Advocates of the various psychosocial interventions have typically posited that their respective approaches confer reduced risk, either by virtue of altering predisposing mechanisms involved in the causal chain producing future episodes or by virtue of providing long-lasting compensatory skills that can be applied by the patient long after treatment is terminated (see, for example, Beck et al. 1979; Becker et al. 1987; Klerman et al. 1984; Rehm 1977).

As described in an as yet unpublished manuscript by Evans et al., all patients evidencing either partial or full clinical response to 12 weeks of active treatment in the CPT project were followed across a 2-year posttreatment follow-up period. Patients in pharmacotherapy alone had been randomly assigned to either medication withdrawal, beginning at the end of the 12-week active treatment period, or medication continuation, to continue through the end of the 1st year of the 2-year follow-up. (The pharmacotherapy-alone condition had been treated as a double-sized cell from the beginning of the trial to permit sufficient sample sizes to support differential treatment during the follow-up.) Treatment responders in cognitive therapy alone and combined cognitive therapy–pharmacotherapy terminated all subsequent treatment after the 12th-week posttreatment reevaluation interview, meaning that responders in the combined condition were withdrawn from study medications at exactly the same time and in the same manner as responders in the pharmacotherapy with no continuation condition described above. In each instance, medication dosage levels were reduced to 50% of the final maximum treatment dosage at the beginning of week 13 (the 1st follow-up week), and to 0 at the beginning of week 14 (the 2nd follow-up week). Patients in pharmacotherapy alone kept on continuation medications through the 1st year of the 2-year follow-up period were similarly withdrawn from study medications over a 2-week interval at the end of the 1st follow-up year.

All patients returned for a clinical reevaluation with an interviewer blind to prior treatment condition every 6 months. In addition, all patients were asked to complete a mailer including the self-report BDI and inquiries regarding any intercurrent negative life events or non-scheduled treatment on a monthly basis. Any patient evidencing an elevation in syndrome depression on these monthly mailers was asked to come in for a clinical reevaluation within a week. Patients evidencing elevated BDI scores of 16 or above over a 2-week period were considered to have exhibited a clinical relapse. Although we had originally intended to require an elevated HRSD score of 12 or above within this same interval in our relapse criterion, we were not able to get all such patients to return in a timely fashion for clinical interview. Twelve patients met our criterion for a clinical relapse. All 12 evidenced two consecutive elevated BDI scores. Ten of those 12 patients evidenced elevated HRSD scores, whereas the remaining 2 patients did not return for clinical reevaluation in a timely fashion and therefore were not evaluated on the HRSD.

Survivorship analyses were used to evaluate differences in relapse rates among the four treatment conditions (Cox and Oakes 1984; Elandt-Johnson and Johnson 1980; Lee 1980). Survivorship analyses not only consider whether a relapse event has occurred, but also take into consideration the amount of time an individual has gone in follow-up before experiencing that event. Because subsequent status after the initial clinical relapse was likely to be contaminated by further treatment, we chose "time to first relapse" as our best index of posttreatment risk. Similarly, comparisons between the conditions based solely on cross-sectional data would also be contaminated by variability in subsequent postrelapse treatment and would not provide a cumulative assessment of ongoing risk.

Figure 2-5 presents "time to first relapse" as a function of treatment condition. Fifty of the 64 treatment completers evidenced sufficient response to enter the follow-up, 12 each (75%) in the drug–no maintenance, drug plus maintenance, and cognitive therapy conditions, and 14 (88%) in the combined cognitive therapy–pharmacotherapy condition. Six patients were lost to follow-up due to noncompliance with the assessment procedures, two each in drug–no maintenance and cognitive therapy, and one each in drug plus maintenance and combined cognitive therapy–pharmacotherapy. Patients in the medication–no maintenance condition evidenced the greatest rate of relapse, with 5 of 10 (50%) at-risk patients evidencing at least one relapse over the 2-year interval (Figure 2-5). Further, all five of these relapses occurred over the first 4 months. Only 3 of 11 (27%) of the medication plus maintenance patients, 2 of 10 (20%) of the cognitive therapy patients, and 2 of 13 (15%) of the combined cognitive therapy–pharmacotherapy patients evidenced one or more relapses. Further, the bulk of the relapses in the last three conditions occurred later in the follow-up than they did in the drug–no maintenance condition. Survivorship analyses contrasting the drug–no maintenance condition versus the other three conditions pooled indicated a significant preventive effect. Similarly, the specific contrast between drug–no maintenance versus prior cognitive therapy (pooling cognitive therapy alone and combined cognitive therapy–phar-

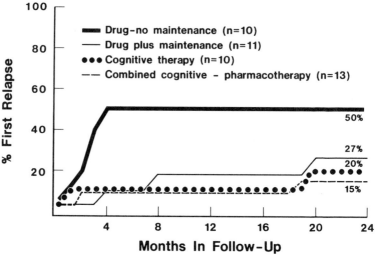

Figure 2-5.   Relapse using conservative criteria (2 consecutive Beck Depression Inventory scores ≥16). Adapted with permission from Hollon et al. 1988.

macotherapy, but excluding medication plus maintenance) was also significant.

This pattern is, of course, indicative of differential prevention, either as a function of ongoing continuation medication or prior cognitive therapy. This finding is wholly consistent with the results obtained in other recent follow-up designs, in which prior cognitive therapy during acute treatment, either alone or in combination with pharmacotherapy, produced subsequent relapse rates lower than those associated with medication that was subsequently withdrawn (Blackburn et al. 1986; Simons et al. 1986). As was previously described, the only follow-up study not evidencing such a finding did evidence a nonsignificant trend, and that in the context of a design that confounded response with relapse, overestimating differences in the former at the expense of underestimating differences in the latter (Kovacs et al. 1981). Further, our CPT data clearly indicated that this differential prevention was not simply a consequence of medication withdrawal, because patients in the combined cognitive therapy–pharmacotherapy condition were withdrawn from medication at the end of active treatment on precisely the same schedule as the pharmacotherapy–no maintenance patients, with no indication of any increment in relapse rates in the former condition. Similarly, the medication continuation patients were withdrawn from medications in precisely the same manner at the end of the 1st year of the 2-year follow-up, after the end of the period of greatest risk for clinical relapse (Beck 1967; Klerman 1978; Prien and Caffey 1977), again with no detectable increment in the rate of relapse. Any tendency to relapse produced solely as a consequence of medication withdrawal should have manifested itself in each of these two conditions. That it did not suggests that increased risk for relapse after medication withdrawal is a function of the presence of independent, temporally linked risk factors not being adequately altered or suppressed, not a "rebound" effect associated with medication withdrawal itself.

Establishing such a preventive effect is, we think, particularly exciting. Clearly, something is changed or something is gained during cognitive therapy that protects patients against subsequent symptomatic relapse (Hollon et al. 1988). Precisely what that something is remains to be determined, but there were indications that it may involve systematic alterations in the way formerly depressed patients generated causal explanations for negative life events.

Although we regard this to be an especially important finding, there is one caveat we need to offer. Although these data suggest a preventive effect for cognitive therapy (or continuation medication) that cannot be explained simply as an artifact of any rebound from medication withdrawal, it is not clear precisely what is being prevented. A distinction can be drawn between symptomatic *relapse*, defined as the return of symptoms associated with the prior episode, versus *recurrence*, the onset of symptoms associated with a wholly new episode (Klerman 1978; Prien and Caffey 1977). As we have argued elsewhere, the risk for symptomatic return after successful pharmacotherapy should be greatest during the interval between the time that remission is induced by successful treatment and the time that the underlying episode would have been expected to take to run its course spontaneously (Hollon et al., in press). The existence of such a "period of risk" is implicit in the growing recognition that pharmacotherapy needs to be extended beyond the time that remission is initially evident (Prien and Kupfer 1986). We (Hollon et al., in press) examined the survivorship curves reported in two major continuation medication trials (Glen et al. 1984; Prien et al. 1984) and found that risk was approximately two to three times as great for the first 6–12 months after pharmacologically induced symptomatic remission than it was for the period that followed. This is exactly what would be expected if patients treated pharmacologically were withdrawn from medications before their underlying episode had run its course; that is, if risk for relapse was independent of and additive with the ongoing risk for recurrence.

What this suggests is that it is premature to claim that cognitive therapy is effective in preventing the onset of new episodes after remission (i.e., recurrences), because the differences observed in our CPT project follow-up were largely the consequence of early symptom return in pharmacologically treated patients withdrawn from medications after 3 months of treatment, well within any period of risk for relapse associated with the treated episode. Although we do think that the CPT project demonstrates a preventive effect (as do the previous Blackburn et al. [1986] and Simons et al. [1986] reports), we think this effect was largely determined by the prevention of differential relapse, not recurrence. That is not to say that cognitive therapy might not prevent the onset of wholly new episodes; it is reasonable to infer that if a therapy can prevent symptomatic relapse it might also prevent symptomatic recurrence. However, our follow-up design, in which patients were initially withdrawn from medications during the period of risk for relapse, was simply not adequate for detecting the prevention of differential recurrence. Because we did withdraw the drug plus maintenance patients from medication at the beginning of the 2nd year of the 2-year follow-up, the contrast between those patients and the patients who had received prior cognitive therapy should indeed have been informative about differential recurrence. There were no detectable differences between those groups of patients across the 2nd year of the follow-up (Figure 2-5). This would argue against any preventive effect for cognitive therapy with respect to recurrence. However, sample sizes, small to begin with, were even further reduced by prior relapse and attrition, making this a less than ideal test of the differential recurrence hypothesis. Even more important, as we noted earlier, the average intermorbid risk between episodes for patients remitting spontaneously has been estimated to be about 3 years (Beck 1967). This means that the period during which the contrast between drug plus prior maintenance versus prior cognitive therapy would have been informative about differential recurrence (i.e., the 12-month period beginning after the 1st year of the 2-year follow-up) was only about one-third as long as would have been necessary to have allowed maximum design power. Clearly, future studies need to be designed to examine more adequately the potential distinction between the differential prevention of relapse versus recurrence, but any indication of differential prevention is, we believe, a most exciting finding that deserves to be explored further.

Mediation of Change

DeRubeis et al. (in press) attempted to evaluate which components of the respective treatment modalities were most directly associated with observed change and which client mechanisms mediated the changes observed. Of the several cognitive and biological variables examined, only the Attributional Styles Questionnaire (ASQ; Seligman et al. 1979), a measure of explanatory style, evidenced a pattern of greater differential change in cognitive therapy. That is, responders in cognitive therapy or combined cognitive therapy–pharmacotherapy evidenced greater change on this measure than they did in pharmacotherapy alone, despite the fact that change in syndrome depression was as great in that latter condition as it was in cognitive therapy alone. The ASQ is a measure of explanatory style, the way in which people explain the events that happen to them. Prior research has indicated that depressed individuals are more likely to adopt internal, global, stable explanations for negative life events than are nondepressed individuals (Peterson and Seligman 1984). Explanatory style has been proposed as an important predispositional factor in clinical depression (Abramson et al. 1978). Given the specificity of change in ASQ scores evident in DeRubeis et al. (in press) and the differential relapse prevention already described, explanatory style would appear to be a leading candidate as a mediator of cognitive therapy's relapse-prevention effect.

Proportional hazards linear regression models (Cox 1972), with Breslow's (1974) modification for tied data, were used to evaluate potential predictors of relapse prevention. A variety of posttreatment indices were found to predict subsequent relapse. However, when residual posttreatment depression was controlled, only explanatory style, as measured by the ASQ, continued to predict subsequent relapse. Thus, posttreatment explanatory style was predictive of subsequent relapse over and above the prediction provided by residual variability in posttreatment syndrome depression.

We next attempted to evaluate whether ASQ levels could be said to mediate the impact of cognitive therapy on subsequent relapse. Treatment execution had been monitored via independent ratings of session audiotapes on two measures: the Minnesota Therapy Rating Scale (DeRubeis et al. 1982), which provides an estimate of the fidelity of adherence to cognitive therapy and the quality of the therapeutic relationship (typically considered to be a nonspecific component of treatment), and the Cognitive Therapy Scale, a measure developed by Young and Beck, which provides a measure of the quality of the execution of cognitive therapy. We generated a combined index of the quality of execution of cognitive therapy and an index of the quality of the therapeutic relationship from these two measures. Both indices significantly predicted subsequent relapse.

We next conducted a regression-based path analysis to determine whether explanatory style could be said to mediate the preventive impact of cognitive therapy on subsequent relapse. According to Baron and Kenny (1986), three conditions must be met in order to reject the hypothesis that the relation between explanatory style and subsequent relapse is purely epiphenomenal. First, the potential mediator itself should be significantly predicted by the independent variable. In fact, when posttreatment attributional style was regressed on the quality of cognitive therapy variable, the relation was indeed significant. Second, the independent variable should significantly predict the dependent variable (subsequent relapse) when the purported mediator is not considered. As previously noted, the quality of execution of cognitive therapy did indeed predict subsequent relapse. Finally, the relation between the dependent variable, clinical relapse, and the purported mediator, explanatory style (as measured by the ASQ), must be significant when the dependent variable is regressed simultaneously on both the mediator and the independent variable, quality of execution of cognitive therapy. Once again, this relation was significant. If the covariation between posttreatment explanatory style and subsequent relapse had been merely epiphenomenal (i.e., the consequence of third-variable causality), it should not have passed this third test. We should also note that although the quality of the therapeutic relationship also predicted subsequent relapse, it did not appear that this relation was mediated through explanatory style, as was the case for the quality of execution of the cognitive therapy–specific components of the larger treatment package. These data indicate that explanatory style, as measured by the ASQ, appears to be a causal mediator (or, at the least, a marker for a causal mediator) with respect to cognitive therapy's preventive effect on subsequent relapse.

CONCLUSIONS

Overall, we think that the available literature, including our own recently completed CPT project, suggests that combined cognitive therapy–pharmacotherapy provides the benefits of either single modality while compensating for the limitations of each. Combined treatment appears to be at least the equal of, and possibly superior to, either single modality in terms of acute response (whether defined in terms of the average magnitude or the universality of that response), comparably acceptable to either alone, and as capable of preventing subsequent relapse as the best of the single modalities. The only evaluative dimension on which it might prove to be less desirable than either of the single modalities is that of safety; the risk of undesirable side effects and the availability of a potentially lethal substance may prove to be greater in the combined treatment than in cognitive therapy alone, although that remains an open question. Although there were few indicators of differential response, those that did emerge suggest that the search for specific indicators to particular drug-psychotherapy combinations might be fruitful.

The indication that cognitive therapy may prevent subsequent relapse, whether presented alone or in combination with medications, is particularly exciting. Further, the indication that this effect might be mediated by specific changes in explanatory style is particularly important theoretically. Such indications may point the way to strategies that are truly preventive in nature, perhaps even applicable to individuals who are at elevated risk but who have not yet experienced their first episode of depression. Further work is clearly indicated in this regard. At this time, however, it does appear that combined cognitive therapy–pharmacotherapy may ultimately prove to best maximize both response and relapse prevention relative to either single modality alone.

REFERENCES

Abramson LY, Seligman MEP, Teasdale JD: Learned helplessness in humans: critique and reformulation. J Abnorm Psychol 87:49–74, 1978

Baron RM, Kenny DA: The moderator-mediator variable distinction in social psychological research: conceptual, strategic, and statistical considerations. J Pers Soc Psychol 51:1173–1182, 1986

Beck AT: Depression: Clinical, Experimental, and Theoretical Aspects. New York, Harper & Row, 1967

Beck AT, Ward CH, Mendelson M, et al: An inventory for measuring depression. Arch Gen Psychiatry 4:561–571, 1961

Beck AT, Rush AJ, Shaw BF, et al: Cognitive Therapy of Depression. A Treatment Manual. New York, Guilford, 1979

Beck AT, Hollon SD, Young JE, et al: Treatment of depression with cognitive therapy and amitriptyline. Arch Gen Psychiatry 42:142–148, 1985

Becker RE, Heimberg RG, Bellack AS: Social Skills Training Treatment for Depression. New York, Pergamon, 1987

Bellack AS, Hersen M, Himmelhoch J: Social skills training compared with pharmacotherapy and psychotherapy in the treatment of unipolar depression. Am J Psychiatry 138:1562–1567, 1981

Bielski RJ, Friedel RO: Prediction of tricyclic antidepressant response: a critical review. Arch Gen Psychiatry 31:1479–1489, 1976

Blackburn IM, Bishop S, Glen AIM, et al: The efficacy of cognitive therapy in depression: a treatment trial using cognitive therapy and pharmacotherapy, each alone and in combination. Br J Psychiatry 139:181–189, 1981

Blackburn IM, Eunson KM, Bishop S: A two-year naturalistic follow-up of depressed patients treated with cognitive therapy, pharmacotherapy and a combination of both. J Affective Disord 10:67–75, 1986

Breslow NE: Covariance analysis of censored survival data. Biometrics 30:89–99, 1974

Carroll BJ, Feinberg M, Greden JF, et al: A specific laboratory test for the diagnosis of melancholia. Arch Gen Psychiatry 38:15–22, 1981

Cohen J: Statistical Power Analysis for the Behavioral Sciences. New York, Academic, 1969

Covi L, Lipman RS: Cognitive-behavioral group psychotherapy combined with imipramine in major depression. Psychopharmacol Bull 23:173–176, 1987

Covi L, Lipman RS, Derogatis LR, et al: Drugs and group psychotherapy in neurotic depression. Am J Psychiatry 131:191–197, 1974

Cox DR: Regression models with life tables (with discussion). Journal of the Royal Statistical Society of Britain 34:187–220, 1972

Cox DR, Oakes D: Analysis of Survival Data. London, Chapman & Hall, 1984

DeRubeis RJ, Hollon SD, Evans MD, et al: Can psychotherapies for depression be discriminated? A systematic investigation of cognitive therapy and interpersonal psychotherapy. J Consult Clin Psychol 50:744–756, 1982

DeRubeis RJ, Evans MD, Hollon SD, et al: How does cognitive therapy work? Cognitive change and symptom change in cognition therapy and pharmacotherapy for depression. J Consult Clin Psychol (in press)

Elandt-Johnson RC, Johnson NL: Survival Models and Data Analysis. New York, John Wiley, 1980

Elkin I, Shea T, Watkins J, et al: NIMH Treatment of Depression Collaborative Research Program. Presented at the 17th annual meeting of the Society for Psychotherapy Research, Wellesley, MA, June 19, 1986

Endicott J, Spitzer RL: A diagnostic interview: the Schedule for Affective Disorders and Schizophrenia. Arch Gen Psychiatry 35:837–844, 1978

Friedman AS: Interaction of drug therapy with marital therapy in depressed patients. Arch Gen Psychiatry 32:619–637, 1975

Garfield SL: Research on client variables in psychotherapy, in The Handbook of Psychotherapy and Behavior Change, 2nd Edition. Edited by Garfield SL, Bergin AE. New York, John Wiley, 1978, pp 191–232

Garvey MJ, Hollon SD, Evans MD, et al: The association of MHPG to dexamethasone suppression test status. Psychiatry Res 24:223–230, 1988

Glassman AH, Perel JM, Shostak M, et al: Clinical implications of imipramine plasma levels for depressive illness. Arch Gen Psychiatry 34:197–204, 1977

Glen AIM, Johnson AL, Shepherd M: Continuation therapy with lithium and amitriptyline in unipolar depressive illness: a randomized, double-blind controlled trial. Psychol Med 14:37–50, 1984

Gram LF, Reisby N, Ibsen I, et al: Plasma levels and anti-depressant effect of imipramine. Clin Pharmacol Ther 19:318–324, 1976

Hamilton M: A rating scale for depression. J Neurol Neurosurg Psychiatry 23:56–62, 1960

Hathaway SR, McKinley JC: The Minnesota Multiphasic Personality Inventory Manual. New York, Psychological Corporation, 1951

Hollon SD: Comparisons and combinations with alternative approaches, in Behavior Therapy for Depression. Edited by Rehm LP. New York, Academic, 1981, pp 33–71

Hollon SD, Beck AT: Psychotherapy and drug therapy: comparisons and combinations, in The Handbook of Psychotherapy and Behavior Change, 2nd Edition. Edited by Garfield SL, Bergin AE. New York, John Wiley, 1978, pp 437–490

Hollon SD, Evans MD, DeRubeis RJ: Preventing relapse following treatment for depression: the Cognitive Pharmacotherapy Project, in Stress and Coping Across Development. Edited by Field T, McCabe P, Schneiderman N. Hillsdale, NJ, Lawrence Erlbaum, 1988, pp 227–243

Hollon SD, Evans MD, DeRubeis RJ: Cognitive mediation of relapse prevention following treatment for depression: implications of differential risk, in Psychological Aspects of Depression. Edited by Ingram RE. New York, Plenum (in press)

Horowitz LM, Inouye D, Siegelman EY: On averaging judges' ratings to increase their correlation with an external criteria. J Consult Clin Psychol 47:453–458, 1979

Jacobson NS, Follette WC, Revenstorf D: Psychotherapy outcome research: methods for reporting variability and evaluating clinical significance. Behavior Therapy 15:336–352, 1984

Klein DF, Davis JM: Diagnosis and Drug Treatment of Psychiatric Disorders. Baltimore, MD, Williams & Wilkins, 1967

Klerman GL: Long-term treatment of affective disorders, in Psychopharmacology: A Generation of Progress. Edited by Lipton MA, DiMascio A, Killam KF. New York, Raven, 1978, pp 187–213

Klerman GL: Drugs and psychotherapy, in The Handbook of Psychotherapy and Behavior Change, 3rd Edition. Edited by Garfield SL, Bergin AE. New York, John Wiley, 1986, pp 777–818

Klerman GL, DiMascio A, Weissman M, et al: Treatment of depression by drugs and psychotherapy. Am J Psychiatry 131:186–191, 1974

Klerman GL, Rounsaville B, Chevron E, et al: Manual for Short-term Interpersonal Psychotherapy (IPT) of Depression. New York, Basic Books, 1984

Kovacs M, Rush AJ, Beck AT, et al: Depressed outpatients treated with cognitive therapy or pharmacotherapy. Arch Gen Psychiatry 38:33–39, 1981

Lavori PW, Keller MB, Klerman GL: Relapse in affective disorders: a reanalysis of the literature using life table methods. J Psychiatr Res 18:13–25, 1984

Lee ET: Statistical Methods for Survival Data Analysis. Belmont, CA, Lifetime Learning Publication, 1980

Ling W, Dorus W, Hargreaves WA, et al: Alternative induction and crossover schedules for methadylacetate. Arch Gen Psychiatry 41:193–199, 1984

McLean PD, Hakstian AR: Clinical depression: comparative efficacy of outpatient treatments. J Consult Clin Psychol 47:818–836, 1979

Morris JB, Beck AT: The efficacy of antidepressant drugs: a review of research (1958–1972). Arch Gen Psychiatry 30:667–674, 1974

Murphy GE, Simons AD, Wetzel RD, et al: Cognitive therapy and pharmacotherapy, singly and together in the treatment of depression. Arch Gen Psychiatry 41:33–41, 1984

Paul GL: Outcome research in psychotherapy. J Consult Psychol 31:109–118, 1967

Peterson C, Seligman MEP: Causal explanations as a risk factor in depression: theory and evidence. Psychol Rev 91:347–374, 1984

Prien RF, Caffey EM: Long-term maintenance drug therapy in recurrent affective illness: current status and issues. Diseases of the Nervous System 164:981–992, 1977

Prien RF, Kupfer DJ: Continuation drug therapy for major depressive episodes: how long should it be maintained? Am J Psychiatry 143:18–23, 1986

Prien RF, Kupfer DJ, Mansky PA, et al: Drug therapy in the prevention of recurrences in unipolar and bipolar affective disorders. Arch Gen Psychiatry 41:1096–1104, 1984

Prusoff BA, Weissman MM, Klerman GL, et al: Research diagnostic criteria subtypes of depression: their role as predictors of differential response to psychotherapy and drug treatment. Arch Gen Psychiatry 37:796–801, 1980

Raskin A, Schulterbrandt JG, Reatig N, et al: Differential response to chlorpromazine, imipramine, and placebo. Arch Gen Psychiatry 23:164–173, 1970

Rehm LP: A self-control model of depression. Behavior Therapy 8:787–804, 1977

Rosenbaum M: A schedule for assessing self control behaviors: preliminary findings. Behavior Therapy 11:109–121, 1980

Roth D, Bielski R, Jones M, et al: A comparison of self-control therapy and combined self-control therapy and antidepressant medication in the treatment of depression. Behavior Therapy 13:133–144, 1982

Rounsaville BJ, Klerman GL, Weissman MM: Do psychotherapy and pharmacotherapy for depression conflict? Arch Gen Psychiatry 38:24–29, 1981

Rush AJ, Beck AT, Kovacs M, et al: Comparative efficacy of cognitive therapy and pharmacotherapy in the treatment of depressed outpatients. Cognitive Therapy and Research 1:17–37, 1977

Rush AJ, Hollon SD, Beck AT, et al: Depression: must pharmacotherapy fail for cognitive therapy to succeed? Cognitive Therapy and Research 2:199–206, 1978

Seligman MEP, Abramson LY, Semmel A, et al: Depressive attributional style. J Abnorm Psychol 88:242–247, 1979

Simons AD, Lustman PJ, Wetzel RD, et al: Predicting response to cognitive therapy of depression: the role of learned resourcefulness. Cognitive Therapy and Research 9:79–89, 1985

Simons AD, Murphy GE, Levine JE, et al: Cognitive therapy and pharmacotherapy for depression: sustained improvement over one year. Arch Gen Psychiatry 43:43–49, 1986

Spitzer RL, Endicott J: A Diagnostic Interview: Schedule for Affective Disorders and Schizophrenia (SADS), 3rd Edition. New York, Biometrics Research, New York State Psychiatric Institute, 1979

Spitzer RL, Endicott J, Robins E: Research Diagnostic Criteria: rationale and reliability. Arch Gen Psychiatry 35:773–782, 1978

Spitzer RL, Endicott J, Robins E: Research Diagnostic Criteria (RDC) for a Selected Group of Functional Disorders, 3rd Edition. New York, Biometrics Research, New York State Psychiatric Institute, 1979

Teasdale JD, Fennell MJV, Hibbert GA, et al: Cognitive therapy for major depressive disorder in primary care. Br J Psychiatry 144:400–406, 1984

Uhlenhuth EH, Lipman RS, Covi L: Combined pharmacotherapy and psychotherapy: controlled studies. J Nerv Ment Dis 148:52–64, 1969

Weissman MM, Prusoff BA, DiMascio A, et al. The efficacy of drugs and psychotherapy in the treatment of acute depression episodes. Am J Psychiatry 136:555–558, 1979

Zis AP, Goodwin FK: Major affective disorder as a recurrent illness: a critical review. Arch Gen Psychiatry 36:835–839, 1979

Chapter 3

Group Psychotherapy and Pharmacotherapy of Depression

Lino Covi, M.D.
Ronald S. Lipman, Ph.D.
James E. Smith II, M.D.

Chapter 3

Group Psychotherapy and Pharmacotherapy of Depression

Among the current modalities of treatment for depression, the combination of group psychotherapy and pharmacotherapy is very frequently employed. However, in the extensive clinical literature on group psychotherapy accumulated since 1906, few discussions of its use with depressive patients can be found. Slavson (1955) listed depression among the contraindications for group therapy, but noted that "many patients included in this category of counter-indications can be treated in group provided they also receive parallel individual treatment" (p. 21). As Hollon and Shaw pointed out, this position appears related to the concern that depressive patients would not only fail to benefit from the group, but would impede the therapeutic process of the group as a whole as well as due to their "self absorption, unrelieved pessimism, desires for immediate symptom relief, and rejection of others' symptoms" (1979, p. 329). Wolf (1967) noted that patients falling in the excluded categories have been found to benefit from group therapy when assigned to homogeneous groups whose members suffer from the same problem.

These concepts about suitability for group psychotherapy were derived from a view of this modality as most effective for characterologic problems (Slavson 1955). Yalom (1970) sees diagnostic classification as not relevant to group work and subsumes depression into the categories of neurotic and characterologic problems where the goal of group psychotherapy would be building new defenses and changing coping styles and characterologic structure. Of his 11 "core" mechanisms of change, cohesiveness and interpersonal learn-

The studies reported in this chapter were supported by ADAMHA Grants MH-15720 and MH-33585 from the National Institute of Mental Health. Joseph H. Pattison, M.D., David Roth, Ph.D., Laura Primakoff, Ph.D., Vincent Greenwood, Ph.D., and Norman Epstein, Ph.D., participated as therapists in the studies described.

ing were seen as the most important. With the renewed interest in nosology and the development of behavior and cognitive therapies in the 1970s, a diagnostically homogeneous composition for group psychotherapy of depression became prevalent (Covi and Primakoff 1988).

The drug treatment of depression was introduced in the late 1950s (Kuhn 1970). Rigorously conducted double-blind clinical trials confirmed the initial impression of effectiveness of the tricyclic antidepressants; the prototype of these drugs, imipramine, was found superior to placebo in only 30 of 40 double-blind trials (Brotman et al. 1987). To identify responders and nonresponders, efforts at finding predictors (Raskin 1968) of drug response led to the development of depressive subtypes (Overall et al. 1966) derived from the Brief Psychiatric Rating Scale. Anxious and retarded subtypes of depression responded differentially to antidepressants and phenothiazines.

In combining two effective therapies, the ideal result is that of potentiation; that is, the response to the combination of treatments is greater than the sum of the individual treatments when used alone. The most common response to combined treatment is reciprocation where the effects of the two treatments combined equals the individual effect of the more potent treatment (Uhlenhuth et al. 1969). The best approach for studying the interactions between treatments is evaluating both treatments separately as well as in combination.

FREE-INTERACTION GROUP PSYCHOTHERAPY COMBINED WITH PHARMACOTHERAPY

Design

To apply the criteria suggested by Uhlenhuth et al. (1969) to the study of the combination of group psychotherapy with antidepressants in the treatment of depression, a study (Covi et al. 1974; Covi et al. 1976; Lipman and Covi 1976) was designed to include the following conditions: 1) psychotherapy plus drug, 2) psychotherapy without drug, 3) drug without psychotherapy, and 4) neither drug nor psychotherapy. For condition 2, an inactive placebo control was used. A second medication, diazepam, was also introduced into the study design to provide for a comparison with a sedative-tranquilizing drug. This design would allow a replication of the reported interaction of depressive subtypes with antidepressant drugs and drugs with a tranquilizing action as reported by Overall et al. (1966). Thus, the design included 1) group psychotherapy with placebo, 2) minimal supportive therapy with placebo, 3) group psychotherapy with imipramine, 4) minimal supportive therapy with imipramine, 5) group psychotherapy with diazepam, and 6) diazepam with minimal supportive therapy. The target population was female outpatients ranging in age from 20 to 50 years presenting nonpsychotic depression of at least moderate severity for at least 2 weeks before screening and with low suicide risk. We aimed at achieving a high degree of homogeneity in level of distress. A 2-week placebo washout preceding onset of active treatment was adopted to further increase such homogeneity and to weed out noncooperative patients. The study was conducted in two Baltimore, Maryland, locations, 7 miles apart: the Johns Hopkins Hospital Phipps Outpatient Department and the Gundry Hospital Outpatient Department. The same treatment and research team saw the research patients at both sites on different weekdays. This design provision facilitated data collection and also allowed for the examination of differential clinic effects when all differences in clinic personnel were eliminated.

After screening, all suitable subjects were assigned to one of two experienced psychiatrists (J.H. Pattison and J.E.S. II), who had practiced outpatient psychiatry for 4 and 13 years, respectively. Both psychiatrists completed their residency training at the Phipps Clinic, where they learned group psychotherapy in the program directed by Jerome Frank, M.D. They saw each patient individually for three visits over a 2-week period while placebo was administered under single-blind conditions; clinical assessment and minimal supportive therapy took place during these three visits. Those patients who were cooperative and still met study entry criteria of at least moderate depression at the end of these initial 2 weeks were randomly assigned to one of the six combinations of three drugs and two types of therapy while continuing with the same treating psychiatrist.

Therapy

The group psychotherapy consisted of 16 weekly, 90-minute sessions in groups of three to nine patients. The therapy procedure was that of free interaction (Frank and Powdermaker 1959) and was psychodynamically oriented. The main themes were those of current reality-oriented problems in the patient's life. Therapists made use of transference-focused interpretations. The opportunity for interpersonal learning was clearly present. The groups were open-ended, with new subjects entering the group as they completed the 2-week placebo washout period, and those patients who completed the 16 weekly sessions leaving the group. To improve group cohesion, the research psychotherapy groups were gradually formed over the 3 months preceding the introduction of the first study subject with outpatients who would have qualified for the study ("core patients").

They underwent most of the research procedures as if they were study subjects. During the study, whenever the size of the group decreased excessively, depressed patients who did not qualify for the study for other than diagnostic reasons were introduced into the group. A third category of "core patients" was represented by those study subjects who deviated from protocol in a serious-enough way to require termination of their status as research subjects. If they had not completed all 16 weekly group sessions, although terminated as study subjects, they were continued in the group in a similar manner to the other two categories of core patients. All core patients were discharged from the group after 16 sessions. Their data were not used in the analyses of the results of the study.

Each group was led by the same psychiatrist with a rare substitution by the principal investigator (L.C.) when the regular treating psychiatrists were ill or on vacation. All group sessions were observed by the same social worker who made ratings and also interviewed each patient-designated significant other at pretreatment and at treatment termination. The patients randomly assigned to minimal treatment also designated a significant other, who was interviewed by one of the two social workers mentioned above. The minimal supportive therapy condition consisted of individual interviews of about 20 minutes held 1 week apart for 2 weeks and every 2 weeks thereafter. In these sessions, symptoms and current stressors were surveyed, improvement and side effects assessed, and study medication dosage adjusted. The group-treated patients were also seen individually by their group therapist. These sessions were held at the same time intervals for the same purpose of adjusting medication and monitoring symptoms, side effects, and stressors. This procedure made it possible to exclude discussion of medication from the group psychotherapy sessions. Thus, the only difference between group psychotherapy and minimal supportive therapy was the group sessions received in the former condition.

Medication was started at two capsules per day at the conclusion of the 2-week placebo washout. This initial daily dosage corresponded to 100 mg of imipramine, 10 mg of diazepam, or two lactose capsules. In the absence of poorly tolerated side effects, the dosage was increased the following week to 150 mg of imipramine, 15 mg of diazepam, or three lactose capsules. The two study psychiatrists were encouraged to maintain that dosage level, but could increase or decrease medication by one unit to achieve optimal clinical response and side-effect control. Thus, the prescribed dosage could range between 100 and 200 mg of imipramine and 10 and 20 mg of diazepam. A count of pills returned at each visit by patients indicated that an average of 125 mg per day of imipramine and 12.5 mg per day of diazepam were actually taken.

Maintenance Treatment

At the end of the 19-week study phase, the patients were globally rated as improved or not improved. If not improved, they were offered nonstudy treatment; if improved, they were assigned to a 12-month maintenance treatment schedule. In this schedule, each medication group was randomly assigned either to continue on the same medication at a maintenance dosage of one-half the first-phase dosage or to a placebo. In the placebo condition, one-half of the group received no pills. The study psychiatrist continued to see these patients every 2 weeks in minimal supportive therapy for three sessions. During those sessions, medication was reduced to the maintenance level. Patients were then seen every 4 weeks for the remainder of the 12-month maintenance treatment phase.

Measures

At the initial screening visit, an intake evaluation was done by a psychiatrist other than the treating psychiatrist. He completed the following ratings:

1. The Raskin Depression Scale (RDS; Raskin et al. 1970), on which three 5-point ratings of verbal report, behavior, and secondary symptoms of depression combined to a range of total possible scores of 3 (no depression) to 15 (extreme depression). A minimum score of 7 was required on the RDS for admission and for retention in the study after the 2-week placebo washout.
2. The Covi Anxiety Scale (CAS; Covi and Lipman 1984), built in parallel to the RDS to similarly evaluate anxiety symptoms.
3. The Brief Psychiatric Rating Scale (BPRS), which was used for a computer-assigned classification of the patients into the anxious, hostile, withdrawn, and agitated subtypes of depression (Overall et al. 1966).
4. A rating of length of the present depressive episode in number of weeks.
5. A count of prior episodes of depression.
6. A rating of the peak of illness specifying the point of highest distress during the present episode. A 7-point scale ranging from less than a week to more than a year from intake was used.
7. History of treatment with medication or electroconvulsive therapy.

8. A rating of the patient's attitude toward possible assignment to group therapy on a 5-point scale from very eager to very reluctant.

In addition, data were collected at intake on demographic variables such as age; marital status (three classes); present occupation (seven categories), education, and occupation of head of the household using the Hollingshead manual (Hollingshead 1957); employment history of the patients in four classes; and longest period of employment in lifetime (in months). The patient was also asked to designate a significant other to be interviewed.

At the first visit, after patient assignment, the treating psychiatrist completed the RDS and CAS and made global ratings of patient mood on a 10-cluster scale derived from the Psychiatric Outpatient Mood Scale (POMS) of McNair and Lorr (1964). He also estimated the patient's intelligence on a 7-point scale and attitude toward group therapy and study medication on a 5-point scale. The RDS and CAS were repeated at treatment visit 3, after 2 weeks on placebo, at which point a minimum score of 7 on the RDS was required for study entry. The RDS and CAS were also completed at the last visit for that patient, whether at the end of the 16-week treatment phase or at an earlier termination period when possible. These anxiety and depression ratings were also completed after the biweekly individual interviews held with each patient during the active treatment phase, which followed the first 5 weekly individual sessions. The treating psychiatrist also rated global improvement on a 7-point scale, from very much better to very much worse, at all individual visits, both during placebo washout and after study medications were administered. At every visit, the patient completed a similar global improvement scale, the POMS, and the 58-item, 4-point Hopkins Symptoms Checklist (HSCL; Williams et al. 1968). Two factor solutions were available from the HSCL: a "general" and a "depressed" patient factor solution. The rating time frame of clinical status was "the last several days, including today."

At the second visit, the patient also rated the treating psychiatrist on the Barrett-Lenard Relationship Inventory (RI; Barrett-Lenard 1962), which was scored for the dimensions of level of regard, empathic understanding, unconditionality of regard, and congruence. At the beginning and at the end of the initial active treatment phase, the patient also rated his or her designated significant other on the same RI scale. Although the RI was developed for describing the relationship between therapist and patient, we felt that it could also be used to describe a close relationship such as that with a husband or significant other.

The social worker who also served as a group observer interviewed the patient-designated significant other at the beginning and end of treatment and rated his or her attitude toward mental illness and psychiatric treatment on a 5-point scale from very favorable to very unfavorable. The significant other completed the RI describing his or her relationship with the patient at the pretreatment and posttreatment interviews with the social worker. He or she also rated the general improvement of the patient at the end of the study on a 7-point global improvement scale.

Results

Three hundred forty-six patients were screened for the study; 279 were accepted and 218 were entered into the active treatment phase. Seven percent of the dropouts before active treatment (visit 3 with the treating psychiatrist) had an after-placebo-washout score of less than 7 on the RDS, whereas 23% deviated by taking nonstudy medications and 4% deteriorated and required immediate nonstudy treatment. The remainder of the 2-week washout period dropouts were no-shows or had various logistical problems or personal objections to their treatment assignment.

One hundred forty-nine patients completed the full 16-week active treatment phase with adequate adherence to protocol. Nineteen patients were terminated early because of clinical worsening. Of these 19 patient attritions, 9 patients were taking diazepam, 9 placebo, and 1 imipramine ($\chi^2 = 6.92$, df 2; $P < .05$). The remainder deviated from the medication requirements of the study or failed to keep scheduled appointments (i.e., were no-shows). As mentioned earlier, several of these deviators were continued as members of a psychotherapy group, following much the same procedures as regular study patients. For all study subjects, the last valid visit for use in data analysis was determined retrospectively by careful review of study records by the principal investigator, who was blind to medication assignment. In this regard, 212 patients completed at least 2 weeks of treatment beyond the placebo washout period. These patients had an average of 11 weeks of valid data.

The average age of the accepted patients was 34.4 years, and the typical patient was a white woman (100%), married (71%), Protestant (50%), nonworking (60%), of social class IV (39%). Forty percent of the patients were in their first depressive episode, 28% in their second, and 19% in their third. The Hopkins and Gundry populations differed mainly in social class (Gundry higher), attitude toward drug treatment (Gundry more favorable), longest period of employment (Gundry larger), and duration of medication in the year preceding the study (Gundry longer).

Side-effects of the medications were modest and did not require the removal of patients from the study, being mainly drowsiness and fatigue for diazepam and dry mouth for imipramine.

The study hypotheses were for both active medications to be superior to placebo, for group psychotherapy to be more effective than minimal therapy, and for anxious depressions to respond better to diazepam and withdrawn depressions to respond better to imipramine.

Drug effects. In all analyses, imipramine was found to be more effective than diazepam or placebo. The patients' self-rated global improvement ratings at termination of treatment, after 16 weeks for the completers and after 2 weeks or longer for the noncompleters, showed a lower level of distress for treatment with imipramine compared with diazepam or placebo that was significant by t tests at $P < .002$ (Table 3-1).

Covariance analyses for the 149 completers, using visit 3 pretreatment scores as covariate on patients' self-rated measures, showed a consistent superiority of treatment with imipramine over placebo and over diazepam, whereas diazepam was not significantly different from placebo (Table 3-2). These results were confirmed by end-point analyses performed with all patients who completed at least 2 weeks of treatment (completers and noncompleters). Analyses of covariance with tests for each of the three main effects (medication, type of therapy, and clinic) and tests for interactions among variables are shown in Table 3-3.

In addition to these analyses, a clinical judgment was made at the end of the active initial phase of treatment regarding whether the patient was sufficiently improved clinically to enter a prolonged

Table 3-1.   Patients' mean global improvement ratings

		Imipramine		Placebo		Diazepam	
Patient status	N	n	Mean rating[a]	n	Mean rating[a]	n	Mean rating[a]
Completed 16 weeks	149	51	1.19	43	1.77	55	2.05
Terminated early[b]	63	19	2.16	27	2.70	17	2.53
Total	212	70	1.46	70	2.13	72	2.15

[a]Scale: 0 = very much better, 1 = quite a bit better, 2 = a little bit better, 3 = no change, 4 = a little worse, 5 = quite a bit worse, 6 = very much worse.
[b]Includes all patients who did not complete the 16-week active treatment phase, but did stay on medication at least 2 weeks.
Source.   Reprinted from Covi et al. 1974, p 196. Copyright 1974, The American Psychiatric Association. Reprinted by permission.

maintenance treatment phase that would require either lower active medication dosage or placebo and less frequent physician contact. A reliably higher proportion of patients treated with imipramine (89%) versus diazepam (73%) and placebo (78%) were judged well enough to enter the 12-month maintenance phase of treatment. Further, of the imipramine-treated patients who completed maintenance treatment, those continued on imipramine (n = 24) did significantly better than those switched from imipramine to placebo.

Table 3-2. Summary of P values for Newman-Keuls multiple range tests of patient (completers only) self-rated outcome measures (week 19)

Criterion measure	Imipramine vs. placebo	Imipramine vs. diazepam	Diazepam vs. placebo
HSCL factors			
General sample			
Depression	.01	.01	NS
Anxiety	.05	.10	NS
Obsessive-compulsiveness	.01	.01	.10
Interpersonal sensitivity	.01	.01	NS
Somatization	.05	.01	NS
Depressed sample			
Depression	.01	.01	NS
Anxiety—somatic	.05	.05	NS
Anxiety—phobic	.10	.05	NS
Hostility	.10	.05	NS
Modified POMS factors			
Depression	.01	.01	NS
Hostility	.01	.01	NS
Fatigue	.01	.01	NS
Friendliness	.05	.05	NS
Anxiety	.01	.01	NS
Activity	.01	.01	NS
Well-being	.05	.05	NS
Cognition	NS	.01	.10
Carefreeness	.01	.01	NS

Note. Data were missing for 7 of the 149 patients who completed 16 weeks of active treatment. HSCL = Hopkins Symptom Checklist. POMS = Psychiatric Outpatient Mood Scale.

Table 3-3. Summary of analysis of covariance on outcome measures at week 19 and at end point

| | Patients who completed week 19 (n = 146) | | | | | | | End point of treatment (n = 207) | | | | | | |
| | Drug effects | | | Additional effects | | | | Drug effects | | | Additional effects | | | |
Criterion measure	F	df	P	Source	F	df	P	F	df	P	Source	F	df	P
HSCL factors														
General sample														
Somatization	3.97	2	.02	D×C	3.52	2	.03	4.00	2	.02	D×C	3.34	2	.04
Depression	12.20	2	.0001	D×C	7.66	2	.001	12.55	2	.0001	D×C	4.74	2	.01
Anxiety	3.15	2	.04	D×R$_x$	2.62	2	.07	1.88	2	NS				
Obsessive-compulsiveness	11.10	2	.0001	D×C	4.18	2	.02	8.67	2	.0005				
Interpersonal sensitivity	7.42	2	.001	D×C	4.15	2	.02	10.19	2	.0002	D×C	3.68	2	.03
Depressed sample														
Depression	12.73	2	.0001	D×C	7.19	2	.001	13.04	2	.0001	D×C	4.31	2	.01
Anxiety—somatic	3.54	2	.03					4.23	2	.02	D×R$_x$	3.21	2	.04
Anxiety—phobic	4.13	2	.02					2.84	2	.06				
Hostility	3.78	2	.02	D×C	3.72	2	.03	4.07	2	.02	D×C	3.90	2	.02
Sleep disturbance	1.14	2	NS	D×C	2.08	2	.13	1.33	2	NS	D×R$_x$	5.84	2	.004

Modified POMS factors

Factor	F	df	p	Source	F	df	p	F	df	p	Source	F	df	p
Depression	11.62	2	.0001	D×C	6.95	2	.002	12.66	2	.0001	D×C	4.19	2	.02
Friendliness	4.40	2	.01	D×R$_x$×C	4.99	2	.008	3.63	2	.03	D×C	3.32	2	.04
Anxiety	9.76	2	.0003	D×C	5.06	2	.008	11.39	2	.0001				
Guilt	2.74	2	.07					4.24	2	.02				
Hostility	11.87	2	.0001	D×C	6.18	2	.003	12.60	2	.0001	D×C	5.22	2	.006
Activity	8.45	2	.0006	C	3.83	1	.05	8.24	2	.0006				
Fatigue	10.65	2	.0002	D×C	8.96	2	.0004	8.29	2	.0006	D×C	5.95	2	.004
Well-being	3.53	2	.03					5.58	2	.005	D×C	2.85	2	.06
Cognition	4.96	2	.009	D×R$_x$	3.36	2	.04	3.95	2	.02	D×R$_x$	3.21	2	.04
Carefreeness	6.01	2	.004	C	4.09	1	.04	7.34	2	.001	D×C	3.06	2	.05

D = drug treatment. C = clinic. R$_x$ = type of therapy. HSCL = Hopkins Symptom Checklist. POMS = Psychiatric Outpatient Mood Scale.

Differences in medication effects were found at the two clinics in spite of use of the same research team in both settings. These differences were unexpected and primarily involved diazepam and placebo. Whereas both active medications were superior to placebo at Hopkins, at Gundry, diazepam produced less improvement than placebo (Figure 3-1). This was true for the HSCL factors of depression and somatization. The hostility factor showed no difference between placebo and imipramine, but diazepam had the worst outcome, indicating the possibility of a benzodiazepine hostility effect (Gardos et al. 1968). The larger drug differences found at Gundry are typified by the outcome pattern shown in Figure 3-1. This finding may be related to the more positive attitude toward drug treatment found in Gundry patients.

Psychotherapy effects. Group psychotherapy advantages were generally very limited. Only two patient self-ratings in the end-point analyses revealed an advantage for group therapy: the hostility factor of the HSCL and the anxiety factor of the POMS ($P = .03$). Completer analyses revealed no advantages for either psychosocial intervention, and no advantages for either therapy were found on any of the depression or global improvement ratings. Differences were not apparent at early evaluations.

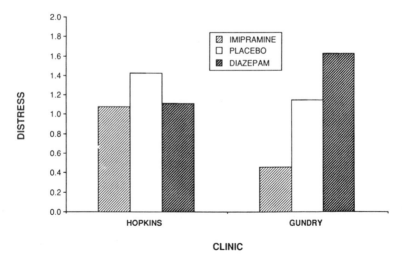

Figure 3-1.   Adjusted mean depression levels at week 19 by Psychiatric Outpatient Mood Scale. Hopkins = Johns Hopkins Hospital Phipps Outpatient Department. Gundry = Gundry Hospital Outpatient Department.

Interestingly, however, a 16-week reliable main effect favoring group psychotherapy was found on the dimension of empathic understanding ($P = .05$) and a trend was found on congruence ($P = .07$) and the total score ($P = .06$) of the RI. Patients in the minimal supportive contact condition perceived their husband or husband-equivalent less positively than did patients assigned to group psychotherapy.

One of the reasons that group psychotherapy effects were not clearly superior to minimal therapy related to the generally strong therapeutic effect of imipramine in both therapy conditions. Thus, imipramine-treated patients tended to do about as well with either group psychotherapy or brief minimal supportive contact. When imipramine-treated patients were taken out of the data pool and the data were reanalyzed with just placebo- and diazepam-treated patients included, the main effects on global improvement and measure of symptom and mood depression favoring psychotherapy were found to be statistically significant as revealed by analysis of covariance techniques and multivariate analysis procedures. The percentage of outcome variance attributable to group psychotherapy effects, however, was smaller (about 5%) than the percentage of outcome variance attributable to medication effects (12%).

A few interaction effects of group psychotherapy with pharmacotherapy were of interest. The result for somatic anxiety indicates a decided advantage for patients treated with imipramine versus placebo in minimal contact (Figure 3-2). In group psychotherapy, placebo-treated patients improved as much as imipramine-treated patients. Thus, the effect of group psychotherapy on somatic anxiety seems unaided by antidepressants. This finding reminds us of Jones's (1944) success with the use of group techniques in psychosomatic disorders. Similar analyses of doctors' ratings largely paralleled the results of the self-ratings.

Predictor analyses. Multiple regression analyses of 22 predictors of improvement selected on the basis of previous research findings (Covi et al. 1976) revealed eight factors that consistently predicted treatment response on measures of depression, anxiety, and global improvement. These variables were significantly related to treatment outcome in at least one-third of the predictor analyses. Four variables predicted outcome regardless of treatment assignment: 1) initial level of distress: low initial distress predicted low final levels of distress, although patients with high initial distress improved relatively more; 2) drug assignment: imipramine-treated subjects improved substantially more than either diazepam- or placebo-treated subjects; 3) a poor employment history predicted less improvement; and 4) a

positive attitude toward group psychotherapy predicted a good outcome regardless of the actual treatment the patient received, probably
reflecting the influence of stronger motivation for change.

Two predictor variables interacted with medication. Being on
estrogen-replacement therapy or on an estrogen-type contraceptive
resulted in as good a response to diazepam as that obtained with
imipramine, probably reflecting a pharmacologic interaction. A relatively lower intelligence level correlated with a better response to both
active drugs relative to placebo than did a higher intelligence level.

Two predictors interacted with type of therapy. Subjects with a
lower initial distress score on the interpersonal sensitivity factor of the
HSCL (feeling critical of others, feeling inferior) did better in group
therapy, whereas persons high in interpersonal sensitivity did better
in minimal contact, indicating that persons with less interpersonal
difficulties will do better in a type of group therapy where interpersonal learning occurs. The recent National Institute of Mental Health
Treatment of Depression Collaborative Research Program also
revealed that patients who were socially better adjusted responded
better in interpersonal therapy (Elkin et al., personal communication).
Finally, patients whose significant other expressed a negative view of
psychiatric treatment improved more in group than in minimal
supportive therapy, indicating that group psychotherapy may effectively counteract a nonsupportive home environment.

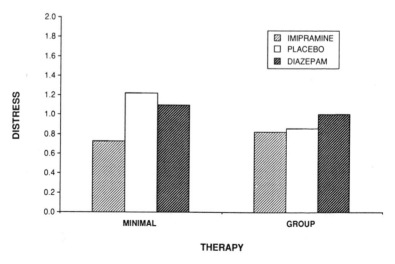

Figure 3-2. Adjusted mean for somatic anxiety levels at week 19.

Subtypes of depression interactions. The four BPRS-derived subtypes of depression did not interact with drugs as expected. Imipramine was found to be the most effective medication in all subtypes. Diazepam was not found to be better than placebo in anxious responders and agitated subtypes, but was found to be much worse than placebo in the hostile subtype. This finding supports the negative effect of diazepam on measures of hostility found in prior covariance analyses.

Discussion

Strong imipramine effects were evident in this study of free-interaction group psychotherapy, but only weak group psychotherapy effects were found. One of the possible explanations for the weak group psychotherapy effects could be an insufficient level of cohesiveness in the groups due to their open-endedness. Thus, new patients entered and others left the group on a frequent basis, possibly disrupting the effectiveness of the group curative factors. A closed group might have been more effective. Another possible improvement in group effectiveness could have derived from the therapist taking a more active role. Of course, a totally different psychotherapeutic technique might also have proven more beneficial.

A few years later, the opportunity for examining these possibilities presented itself when detailed manuals of cognitive-behavior therapy became available (Beck et al. 1979).

COGNITIVE-BEHAVIOR GROUP PSYCHOTHERAPY COMBINED WITH PHARMACOTHERAPY

Design

The design of this study (Covi and Lipman 1987) included 1) cognitive-behavior group psychotherapy alone, 2) cognitive-behavior group psychotherapy with imipramine, and 3) traditional free-interaction group psychotherapy alone. The design was developed to examine the effectiveness of closed cognitive-behavior group psychotherapy alone and combined with imipramine. The control was traditional group psychotherapy of the type used in the earlier trial, but with a closed arrangement and other procedural modifications to parallel the procedures of the cognitive-behavior groups. Besides allowing a partial replication of the first study, it permitted us to examine the question of possible increased effectiveness from closed groups. The traditional group also provided for an appropriate control condition to ensure that the improvement from cognitive groups did not just result from the operation of general group curative factors because these factors would also operate within the traditional groups.

The target population for the study was patients with nonbipolar, nonpsychotic major depressive disorders. Patients had to meet Research Diagnostic Criteria (RDC; Spitzer et al. 1978) for major depression of at least 1 month's duration. They were also required to score at least 20 on the Beck Depression Inventory (BDI; Beck et al. 1961) and at least 14 on the physician-rated 17-item Hamilton Rating Scale for Depression (HRSD; Hamilton 1960). Age limits were 18–70 years, and minimum literacy (about a seventh-grade education level) was required. Patients with bipolar affective disorders, schizophrenia, drug or alcohol abuse, and serious suicide risk were excluded. These entry criteria were verified in a second screening evaluation by an independent evaluator, a highly experienced psychiatrist (J.E.S. II) who did not have access to the intake ratings. All treatment was conducted in the Treatment Assessment Research Unit of the Phipps Psychiatric Outpatient Department of the Johns Hopkins Hospital. Almost all subjects for this study were recruited through advertisements placed in a newspaper. A self-rating list derived from DSM-III criteria for a major depressive episode was printed in the newspaper and mailed back by the applicant. Symptomatic volunteers so recruited are comparable to clinic-referred outpatients (Covi et al. 1980). After two screening interviews, accepted patients were randomly assigned to group therapy and were seen for two 1-hour individual visits by the leader of the assigned group. During these visits, held 1 week apart, the respective cognitive or traditional individual technique was followed after a review of history and symptoms was accomplished and role induction instructions were imparted. A third individual session was held after the first two group sessions to ventilate possible group difficulties and to prevent dropouts. Two group sessions were held during the 3rd and 4th weeks of treatment to intensify the rate of treatment. Minutes of each group session were compiled by an observer or by the therapist and were distributed to each member before every group session so that continuity of sessions was assured.

The patients assigned to the combined cognitive-behavior therapy (CBT) group plus imipramine were seen for drug adjustment by the psychiatrist who conducted the traditional group. In his role as drug adjustor, he saw patients weekly for three visits and then every 2 weeks until the end of the active phase of the study.

On completion of the 14-week group course of treatment, the patients were evaluated by the independent evaluator and judged improved or nonimproved, the latter judgment including HRSD scores being at or above study entry criteria. The nonimproved patients were given four additional individual sessions ("optimization") within the framework and using the respective techniques of each type of therapy. Additionally, for patients in combined treatment, an increased dosage of imipramine was employed. Patients were reevaluated at the end of optimization and were either discharged from the study to a nonstudy treatment if not improved or assigned to a 9-month follow-up phase when clinically appropriate. This phase of treatment consisted of monthly visits with their therapist and reevaluation by the independent evaluator every 3 months. The independent evaluator, blind to treatment assignment, saw the subjects at monthly intervals during the active phase, at which time ratings were done. He also saw any patient whom the therapist felt was deteriorating and in need of alternative treatment. When this happened, a final evaluation was conducted.

Assessments

Doctor ratings. At the initial screening visit, the intake doctor completed the HRSD, with a minimum score of 14 on the first 17 items being required. He also completed the CAS and RDS (Covi and Lipman 1984) and used RDC to evaluate the presence of probable or definite major depressive disorder. RDC were also used to rate the presence or absence of subtypes of depression and predominant mood (Spitzer et al. 1978). A patient's self-rating of at least 20 on the BDI was also required. After receiving an explanation of the research and signing the informed consent form, the accepted subjects were reevaluated by the independent evaluator (J.E.S. II), who was blind to intake ratings. Patients were also screened for the presence or absence of inclusion and exclusion criteria, and the accepted patients were assigned to a random treatment list. The independent evaluator completed the same ratings as the intake doctor and the following additional scales: 1) the Global Assessment Scale from the Schedule for Affective Disorders and Schizophrenia (SADS) (Endicott and Spitzer 1978); 2) the doctors' version of the HSCL-90 (HSCL-90—Dr.), an 11-cluster, 7-point scale in which each cluster contained the items of the corresponding factor of the self-rated HSCL-90; and 3) target symptoms rated on a 5-point scale. Target symptoms were developed jointly by the patient and the doctor during the first interview and were the patient's main or most troublesome symptoms. After the initial evaluation, the independent evaluator reevaluated the subjects at monthly intervals. He also completed a 7-point global improvement scale ranging from very much better to very much worse, as compared with the first visit.

The independent evaluator remained blind to treatment assignment, and the patients were given a memo explaining why they should only discuss improvement and not the type of therapy they were receiving with the independent evaluator. As mentioned above, the independent evaluator did final evaluations whenever the patient terminated treatment or before admission to follow-up.

At individual sessions, which occurred at the beginning and at the end of treatment and during follow-up, the therapists completed the CAS and RDS and target symptom ratings. The pharmacotherapist completed a global improvement scale and a treatment Emergent Symptoms Scale for side effects (Guy and Bonato 1970).

Patient ratings. The BDI (Beck et al. 1961), a widely used 21-item self-rating scale for depression, was completed at each visit. Rush et al. (1977) found it differentially sensitive to CBT versus imipramine treatment. Scores on the BDI range from 0 to 63. Beck et al. characterize scores of 0–9 as "not depressed," 10–15 as "mildly depressed," 16–23 as "moderately depressed," and 24 + as "severely depressed."

The HSCL-90, a self-report checklist designed to measure the more common symptoms of distress experienced by psychiatric outpatients, was completed at each visit. The HSCL-90 is a second-generation version of the HSCL that contains the original well-validated factors of depression, anxiety, somatization, obsessive-compulsiveness, and interpersonal sensitivity plus four newly postulated factors of anger-hostility, phobic anxiety, psychoticism, and paranoid ideation (Derogatis et al. 1973).

Factor analysis by Lipman et al. (1979) has revealed the presence of eight clinically meaningful orthogonal factors that were designated somatization, phobic anxiety, retarded depression, agitated depression, obsessive-compulsiveness, interpersonal sensitivity, anger-hostility, and psychoticism.

At each visit, the patient was asked to rate his or her clinical improvement since the start of treatment on a 7-point scale ranging from "very much better" through "no change" to "very much worse." This measure has proved quite sensitive to treatment effects (Lipman et al. 1965).

An abbreviated version of the Social Adjustment Scale (SAS) was completed at the beginning of treatment and repeated twice during the course of treatment. The SAS was developed by Weissman and Bothwell (1976) to assess how well patients function in their significant relationships with others (e.g., marriage, family) and in certain roles such as work, school, and leisure activities. The SAS is viewed as both a mediating (process) variable and an outcome measure because of the critical importance that social adjustment plays in the theoretical formulations of Frank (1974), on which the "traditional" psychotherapy regimen rests. That is, social effectiveness is viewed by Frank as the sine qua non of his "free-interactive" psychotherapy.

The Dysfunctional Attitude Scale (DAS) was completed at pretreatment and twice during the study. Beck and his coworkers are currently using a 40-item version of the DAS (Weissman 1979). The DAS has been employed as an outcome measure, but it is also central to the theory underlying CBT. For this reason, it is also conceptualized here as a mediating or process variable.

The DAS is seen as analogous to the SAS. That is, change on the DAS is seen as a necessary precondition for the effectiveness of CBT in the same manner as the SAS is seen as central to traditional psychotherapy.

Treatment

Treatment manuals were developed for CBT, traditional therapy, and pharmacotherapy. The first two were published elsewhere (Covi et al. 1982, Covi et al. 1988). We summarize them here.

Role induction. Given the importance of the systematic preparation of the patient for psychotherapy (Hoehn-Saric et al. 1964), we employed a role induction procedure as part of this study. This was accomplished during the initial two individual sessions with the cognitive or the traditional therapist that preceded the first group session. During these sessions, treatment assignment and the schedule of treatment visits were explained, and a memo covering these details was given to the patient. A brief review of clinical history followed, and a list of target symptoms was developed and rated for intensity. In the case of cognitive therapy, didactic explanation of the rationale and techniques of therapy and of the importance of self-help home assignments was followed with the patient being given a copy of *Coping With Depression* by Beck and Greenberg (1974). In the case of traditional therapy, the rationale for free-interaction group psychotherapy was briefly reviewed, with emphasis on the responsibility of the patient for attendance and active participation. The absence of judgmental attitudes on anyone's part was stressed. The importance of sharing any thought of premature termination of treatment with the group was also stressed in this session. It must be noted that these procedural points were also made with the patients assigned to cognitive therapy. In general, the individual cognitive therapy sessions had a much higher level of structure, including preset printed agendas, than the traditional sessions, quite in keeping with the different therapies.

Treatment course—group. In CBT, three phases can be distinguished. The first phase is usually played out in the first group session, because the individual sessions largely cover the development of a therapeutic alliance, instillation of hope, and shaping of a conceptualization of depression and its treatment with the identification of problem areas (target symptoms). The second phase involves the implementation of cognitive-behavior modification procedures and the monitoring of treatment response. This phase was initiated in the second individual session and continued throughout most of the group course. The third phase covered the last two sessions and involved examining termination issues, residual unresolved issues, and prevention of recurrence. All group sessions were of 2 hours' duration. To assure standardization of each session, a written preset group agenda was set up on a flip chart in the group room before the session. The agenda of group session 1 is shown in Table 3-4.

Particular emphasis was put on homework assignments to be performed between sessions. This principle, introduced at the first individual session, was reinforced at every opportunity. Homework compliance should be considered crucial to the outcome in cognitive and behavior therapies (Primakoff et al. 1986). At the initial group session, particular importance was given to the discussion of expectations about group therapy. A grid was drawn on the blackboard, and every member's cognitions and emotions "while coming to group today" were entered. Thus, members were trained in identifying

Table 3-4. Agenda for group session 1

1. Set agenda (preset form)
2. Scan Beck Depression Inventory for critical areas
3. Introduce patients to one another
4. Review ground rules
5. Discuss expectations about group therapy
6. Implement group therapy role induction procedure
7. Develop group cohesion by discussing reasons for attending therapy
8. Ask for feedback about individual session 2
9. Discuss current clinical status
10. Go over "Mastery and Pleasure" (M&P) assignment
11. Discuss personal agenda and the relationship between situation, cognition, and mood (SCM)
12. Assign M&P and SCM monitoring exercise
13. Elicit feedback about session
14. Summarize session

cognitions and related emotions, and group cohesion was built as well.

After the first group session, the session agendas showed little variability and are exemplified by the group session 3 agenda (Table 3-5). At this point, a second flip chart was used to write down the members' individual agendas, whereas the blackboard was used to develop general group techniques such as the Record of Dysfunctional Thoughts (Beck et al. 1979) and, in general, to visually reinforce concepts and techniques.

In each CBT group, but not in traditional groups, a therapist and a cotherapist conducted the therapy. A recorder was present to take notes and to prepare the minutes of the session, which were distributed to the patients at the next meeting. The primary therapist saw all patients of his group individually and at all group sessions conducted an initial and a final go-around that included all patients. The initial go-around consisted of a review of symptoms, setting of personal agendas, and reporting on prior homework assignments. The final go-around included new homework assignments and an evaluation of the session by each patient. The cotherapist looked over the BDI forms for critical problem areas such as suicidal ideation and reviewed written homework assignments brought in by the group members. He or she brought pertinent items from these surveys up for discussion and intervened in the discussion whenever the primary therapist needed a respite or the contribution of additional therapeutic techniques. This role is of great help to the primary therapist, who may become fatigued by this very active role. The interventions of the cotherapist allow the primary therapist to detach and to reflect on ongoing exchanges and to plan new strategies. Presession and postsession treatment conferences between the therapists helped them maintain smoothness in this process of "pass-

Table 3-5. Agenda for group sessions 3–13

1. Set personal agenda (allow for session to review cognitive skills and basic beliefs)
2. Scan Beck Depression Inventory for critical areas
3. Elicit reactions to past group sessions
4. Discuss current clinical status
5. Review homework
6. Discuss personal agenda items and special topics
7. Assign homework
8. Elicit feedback about session
9. Summarize session

ing the group baton." Video and audio recordings of the sessions were reviewed by a consultant (B. Shaw, Ph.D.), who gave feedback concerning the correctness of cognitive-behavior techniques.

The manual developed for traditional therapy was less detailed than the CBT manual (Covi et al., in press). This, of course, is in keeping with the unstructured, psychodynamically oriented, free-interaction character of this therapy. Although closed, the style of this group therapy was fairly similar to that used in the prior free-interaction group psychotherapy study, and the therapist was one of the two psychiatrists who had conducted groups in that study, thus offering a partial replication of one treatment condition. One therapeutic principle of this therapy was that sharing depressive themes would facilitate identification of the group members with each other and promote cohesiveness and clinical improvement. An additional assumption was that conflict with authority inherent in the depressive posture and of a transferential nature could be better dealt with within a group context.

The first phase of therapy, covering sessions 1–4, was evocative-supportive and was intended to promote cohesion, universality, and altruism by way of balanced sharing of symptomatology and aggravating circumstances and insights, and the discussion of emergent themes. The therapist would propose a warm-up topic such as anger, helplessness, or suicide, making sure that every member had the opportunity to comment and that those seeming to resist were brought out by soliciting the opinion of the remaining members. At the end of this phase, a transitional question to the next phase was proposed: "How well do we understand each other's predicament?" Phase 2, covering sessions 5–9 and often 10 and 11 as well, aimed at clarification by way of identification of self-defeating trends as resistance to change. Idiosyncratic perceptions and responses were discussed in order for the patient to better appreciate illness and dysphoria. What is changeable and what is not changeable were considered. At the end of this phase, a traditional therapeutic suggestion was made: "I would like each of you to share with us what you have learned about how you make things worse for yourself." Phase 3, covering sessions 12–15, but often starting at session 10, was an assimilative-reorientational phase intended to utilize new undertakings to initiate a better way of life.

Usually the 2-hour sessions were interrupted by a 10-minute intermission for rest and refreshments. The third individual session, which took place after the second group meeting, had particular significance in traditional therapy because of the nonstructured format of the group. In this session, the patient was able to clarify doubts about or resistances to the group. The role of the therapist was primarily passive, although by preparing the group-session minutes, which were distributed to the members at each successive session, he tangibly demonstrated his involvement in the group.

Treatment course—pharmacotherapy. In the four therapy groups in which imipramine and cognitive therapy were used, treatment was conducted in an identical manner to CBT alone, but in addition, every subject was also seen by the traditional therapist in his capacity as pharmacotherapist. He administered imipramine, open label, 50-mg tablets. The dosage schedule was flexible, starting at 50 mg, but increasing to 100–150 mg within 10 days and then a flexible adjustment up to a maximum of 300 mg per day. Some effort was made to retain patients in the study who exhibited more than mild side effects by allowing some patients to be given a very low dosage of medication during the initial month of treatment. The medication administration sessions were no longer than 20 minutes (except for the first one) and were held once a week for 3 weeks and then every other week for the remainder of the study. When a patient needed optimization at the end of group therapy, the pharmacotherapist also saw the patient biweekly, adjusting the dosage to a higher level. At the end of the active treatment phase, if the patient was going into follow-up, the pharmacotherapist tapered the medication to a maintenance level of about one-half that of the active treatment dosage. At that point, patients were randomly assigned to either continue or discontinue imipramine.

Therapists. The CBT therapists included a psychiatrist (L.C.) with 20 years of experience. His training in CBT included a 2-week training seminar at the Philadelphia Center for Cognitive Therapy, followed by supervised training for 1 year at the same center and 2 years of experience in conducting closed CBT groups in collaboration with a number of trained CBT therapists. Throughout the study, sessions were continuously observed directly or on videotape and critiqued by several experts in CBT. The other CBT therapist was a Ph.D. psychologist (D. Roth) with 9 years of training and experience in treating depressed patients with behavior and cognitive techniques. His training was originally in self-control techniques with Lynn Rehm. His therapeutic approach was expanded and modified to conform to Beck's style, and his therapy was monitored by the study consultants. A prestudy, 15-session group was conducted by the two CBT therapists while developing the CBT treatment manual.

The traditional therapist was a psychiatrist (J.H. Pattison, M.D.) with 17 years of experience who had been one of the group therapists in our previous traditional group psychotherapy study. A senior group therapy expert (E. Ascher, M.D.) observed a prestudy 15-session group and assisted in writing the treatment manual. The observations and consultations continued throughout the study.

The pharmacotherapist role was also filled by the same psychiatrist. He had been a therapist for 12 years in 10 controlled psychopharmacological trials. A manual of procedures for drug administration was also developed and implemented.

Results

Of 458 responses to a newspaper advertisement for depressed volunteers, 240 intake evaluations were done; 120 subjects met study criteria, accepted study induction, and signed an informed consent form. Ninety-two subjects were randomized after the second evaluation into one of three assignments: traditional psychotherapy (three groups), CBT (four groups), and CBT plus imipramine treatment (four groups). Of the 92 patients accepted for the study, 19 patients were dropped after treatment assignment and 3 were excluded for not attending the first group session.

The final sample (after attrition before the first group meeting) consisted of 70 subjects (28 males, 42 females) with a mean age of 43.5 years; 65 were Caucasian, and 44% were married. The study volunteers were well educated: 71.5% had more than 12 years of education, and 42.9% were professionals. Sixty-seven percent had prior treatment for emotional distress, 75.7% had prior episodes of depression, 12.9% had a previous hospitalization for an emotional disorder, and 61.4% had previous psychotropic drug treatment. None of these variables differed reliably by treatment assignment. RDC subtype classifications indicated that 74.3% had a recurrent unipolar major depressive disorder and 57.1% were endogenous.

Twenty-five subjects were initially assigned to traditional group therapy (three groups), 32 to CBT group therapy (four groups), and 33 to CBT plus imipramine (four groups). The study was conducted in two successive treatment cycles providing a summer break. There was a 41% reduction in the proportion of attrition from cycle 1 to cycle 2, probably due to improved intake and other management procedures; there was no significant disproportional treatment-related attrition as tested over the three treatments or as tested by combining the CBT conditions versus the traditional treatment condition (χ^2 = 1.43, df 2, and χ^2 = 1.55, df 1, respectively).

A count of actual imipramine tablets taken indicated an average of 135 mg taken per day at the end of the 1st month, 158 mg per day by month 2, and 176 mg and 185 mg per day at months 3 and 4, respectively. Side effects were within expected limits: 30% experienced drowsiness (17% moderate, none severe), and 86% experienced dry mouth (43% moderate, 13% severe).

Treatment outcome was measured by patient self-ratings (BDI, HSCL-90, and Global Improvement Scale—Patient [Lipman et al. 1965]), and ratings made by the independent evaluator after structured patient interviews (HSCL-90—Dr., Global Improvement Scale—Dr., and HRSD). One-way analyses of covariance were used to test for overall differences among the three groups. The covariate used for doctors' ratings was scored at visit 2, that is, the initial evaluation by the independent evaluator. For patients' self-ratings, the covariate used was scored at visit 3, the first individual therapy session. Posttreatment ratings examined were at visit 5 (the 1st group session), visit 12 (the 7th group session), visit 16 (the 11th group session), and visit 20 (the 15th and last group session). Where overall significant treatment effects were evidenced ($P = .05$), the Newman-Keuls multiple range test was used to examine pairwise differences between each of the three treatment conditions. Analyses performed were of the data collected from patients who adhered to the protocol throughout the 14 weeks of treatment (completers; $n = 53$) and for this group of patients plus an additional 17 patients who deviated from protocol after having attended at least 1 week of group therapy; most of these individuals completed at least 1 month (five sessions) of group therapy. The latter patient group ($n = 70$) was referred to as "end point," and their last valid visit (i.e., last visit completed according to protocol) scores were substituted for any missing scores in all analyses of subsequent time periods.

Patient self-rating. A consistent pattern of findings on the BDI was demonstrated by both groups of subjects (i.e., end point and completers). No significant pretreatment effects were found at baseline. One-way analyses of covariance revealed significant between-group differences at the evaluation periods corresponding to group sessions 11 and 15 (after 8 and 12 weeks of group therapy, respectively). Subsequent range tests disclosed that the CBT conditions did not significantly differ from each other, but did evidence significantly lower BDI scores than the traditional condition.

Table 3-6 presents the posttreatment (at 14-week evaluation) classification of BDI scores for the end-point data. Subjects were designated as remitted (BDI score 0–9), mild to moderately depressed (BDI score 10–23), or severely depressed (BDI score 24 or above). By examining BDI scores in this manner, a clinically meaningful picture of treatment-related improvement can be obtained. Thus, 28 CBT patients from the end-point sample were designated as being clinically euthymic, but only 1 traditional patient (3.6%). This was compared to 51.9% for CBT alone and 60.1% for CBT plus imipramine. These percentages are for the end of active treatment and before the follow-up phase of 8–9 months' duration.

Separate χ^2 analyses conducted on the completer samples also revealed significant differences among the treatment groups favoring the CBT conditions. The data and significant results for the end-point sample on mean BDI total scores are illustrated in Figure 3-3.

Patients receiving CBT alone or CBT plus imipramine also displayed a reliably greater reduction on the HSCL for depression after 11 and 15 group sessions as compared with patients receiving traditional therapy.

The three treatment conditions were also contrasted on the 10 HSCL-90–derived scores. The first 8 scores represent hypothesized clusters of psychopathology, whereas the remaining 2 scores reflected empirically determined depression factors (retarded depression and agitated depression). Nine of the 10 dimensions of the HSCL-90

Table 3-6. Beck Depression Inventory (BDI) end-point data

BDI score	CBT alone	CBT + IMI	Total
0–9	14	14	28
10–23	12	6	18
24+	1	3	4
Total	27	23	50

χ^2 = 2.70, 2 df, P = .26, NS

BDI score	CBT alone	TRAD	Total
0–9	14	1	15
10–23	12	10	22
24+	1	9	10
Total	27	20	47

χ^2 = 17.19, 2 df, P = .0002

BDI score	CBT + IMI	TRAD	Total
0–9	14	1	15
10–23	6	10	16
24+	3	9	12
Total	23	20	43

χ^2 = 15.13, 2 df, P = .0005

Note. CBT = cognitive-behavior therapy. IMI = imipramine. TRAD = traditional therapy.

demonstrated a statistically significant advantage for the CBT conditions versus the traditional condition: depression (Figure 3-4), anxiety (Figure 3-5), obsessive-compulsiveness (Figure 3-6), interpersonal sensitivity, phobic anxiety, sleep difficulties, anger-hostility, retarded depression, and agitated depression. These results, as well as those obtained on the BDI and the global improvement scale, are shown in Table 3-7. These differences tended to appear early in the course of treatment and were sustained throughout treatment. Global Improvement Scale ratings also followed the same general pattern, but were statistically significant only in the completer analyses.

Social adjustment. A series of analyses of variance of the patients' rating of social adjustment showed a fairly general pattern of advantage for those patients receiving CBT alone compared with patients receiving traditional therapy or CBT plus imipramine. The patients' ratings of "social life," for example, showed CBT alone to be superior to traditional therapy by the Newman-Keuls test at group sessions 1, 7, and 15 ($P = .01$, $P = .01$, and $P = .05$, respectively) and CBT to be superior to CBT plus imipramine at group sessions 1 and 7 ($P = .01$).

Independent evaluator ratings. Each patient was interviewed by an independent evaluator who remained blind to the patient's therapy

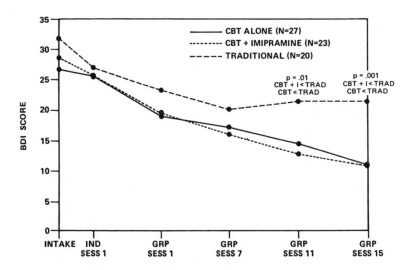

Figure 3-3. Mean Beck Depression Inventory (BDI) total score — end point. CBT = cognitive-behavior therapy. I = imipramine. TRAD = traditional therapy.

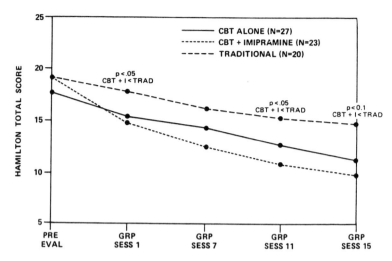

Figure 3-4.   Mean Hamilton Rating Scale for Depression 17-item total score—end point. CBT = cognitive-behavior therapy. I = imipramine. TRAD = traditional therapy.

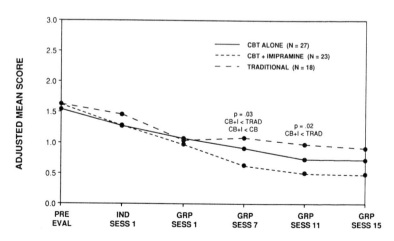

Figure 3-5.   Patient Hopkins Symptom Checklist 90 anxiety factor end point. CBT = cognitive-behavior therapy. I = imipramine. TRAD = traditional therapy.

assignment. The schedule of these interviews was as follows: the first interview was conducted after the intake (screening) visit and before the start of treatment, with the remaining interviews being done at approximately monthly posttreatment intervals (corresponding to group sessions 1, 7, 11, and 15). The independent evaluator rated subjects on the eight HSCL-90 clusters (HSCL-90—Dr.), a 7-point Global Improvement Scale—Dr., and the HRSD.

Independent evaluator ratings were generally consistent with the self-report data. That is, therapeutic advantage for both CBT conditions were seen on the HRSD and several HSCL-90—Dr. dimensions (Table 3-8). Interestingly, the therapeutic advantage of the CBT treatments tended to be detected earlier by the independent evaluator ratings (i.e, at the time of the first group session). This finding seems consistent with the clinical folklore regarding the more rapid detection of changes in depression by observation than by patients' self-reports.

It is also important to note that the independent evaluator ratings reflect a more significant advantage for CBT plus imipramine versus CBT alone and fewer advantages for CBT alone versus traditional therapy (see Table 3-8).

The protocol of the CBT pilot study provided for an optional 1-month optimization phase in which patients could be seen weekly for individual CBT or traditional psychotherapy. The decision to optimize patients who completed their initial 14-week treatment

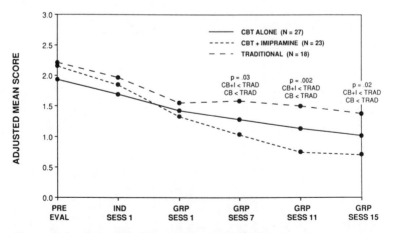

Figure 3-6.   Patient Hopkins Symptom Checklist 90 obsessive-compulsive factor end point. CBT = cognitive-behavior therapy. I = imipramine. TRAD = traditional therapy.

Table 3-7. End-point patient ratings on Hopkins Symptom Checklist 90 (HSCL-90), Beck Depression Inventory, and Global Improvement Scale—Patient

	Means			F	P	Range test P		
	CBT alone	CBT + IMI	TRAD			CBT vs. CBT + IMI	CBT vs. TRAD	CBT + IMI vs. TRAD
HSCL-90 somatization								
Intake	1.03	1.32	1.23	1.159	.32			
Individual session 1	.83	1.07	.98	.772	.47			
Group session 1	.84	.60	.80	1.630	.20			
Group session 7	.75	.46	.66	2.241	.11			
Group session 11	.65	.38	.68	2.278	.11			
Group session 15	.62	.36	.60	1.652	.20			
HSCL-90 obsessive-compulsiveness								
Intake	1.94	2.16	2.22	.719	.49			
Individual session 1	1.70	1.85	1.97	.630	.54			
Group session 1	1.43	1.34	1.56	.787	.46			
Group session 7	1.28	1.04	1.59	3.635	.03*		.05	.01
Group session 11	1.13	.75	1.51	6.826	.002*	.10	.05	.01
Group session 15	1.02	.71	1.38	3.955	.02*		.05	.01
HSCL-90 interpersonal sensitivity								
Intake	1.75	1.65	1.73	.104	.90			
Individual session 1	1.39	1.28	1.35	.136	.87			
Group session 1	1.18	.98	1.23	1.235	.30			
Group session 7	1.00	.76	1.21	3.074	.05*			.01
Group session 11	.90	.60	1.07	4.029	.02*	.05		.01
Group session 15	.77	.57	1.03	3.056	.05*			.01

				F	p			
HSCL-90 depression								
Intake	2.22	2.45	2.68	3.146	.05*			
Individual session 1	1.92	2.05	2.15	.918	.40			
Group session 1	1.46	1.49	1.81	2.022	.14			
Group session 7	1.39	1.11	1.75	4.109	.02*		.10	.01
Group session 11	1.18	.89	1.72	7.131	.002*		.01	.01
Group session 15	1.02	.87	1.55	3.835	.03*		.05	.01
HSCL-90 anxiety								
Intake	1.55	1.63	1.63	.112	.90			
Individual session 1	1.27	1.28	1.46	.497	.61			
Group session 1	1.07	.97	1.04	.183	.83			
Group session 7	.91	.64	1.08	3.899	.03*	.05		.01
Group session 11	.73	.51	.98	3.985	.02*		.10	.01
Group session 15	.72	.49	.91	2.664	.08			
HSCL-90 anger-hostility								
Intake	1.45	1.55	1.09	1.580	.21			
Individual session 1	1.23	1.25	.81	2.049	.14			
Group session 1	.71	.65	.67	.043	.96			
Group session 7	.70	.43	.91	2.667	.08			
Group session 11	.47	.33	.88	4.832	.01*		.01	.01
Group session 15	.38	.30	.65	2.963	.06		.05	.05
HSCL-90 phobic anxiety								
Intake	.58	.65	.82	.649	.53			
Individual session 1	.50	.56	.59	.105	.90			
Group session 1	.41	.32	.36	.553	.58			
Group session 7	.30	.17	.42	3.559	.03*			.01
Group session 11	.25	.14	.41	3.885	.03*			.01
Group session 15	.24	.14	.36	2.000	.14		.10	

Table 3-7. End-point patient ratings on Hopkins Symptom Checklist 90 (HSCL-90), Beck Depression Inventory, and Global Improvement Scale—Patient—Continued

| | Means | | | F | P | Range test P | | |
	CBT alone	CBT + IMI	TRAD			CBT vs. CBT + IMI	CBT vs. TRAD	CBT + IMI vs. TRAD
HSCL-90 sleep								
Intake	2.09	2.39	2.08	.610	.55			
Individual session 1	1.82	1.95	1.81	.112	.89			
Group session 1	1.56	1.05	1.87	5.290	.007*	.05		.01
Group session 7	1.42	.92	1.79	5.466	.006*	.05		.01
Group session 11	1.30	.84	1.43	2.011	.14			
Group session 15	1.12	.79	.78	2.408	.10			
HSCL-90 retarded depression factor								
Intake	2.20	2.29	2.57	1.973	.15			
Individual session 1	1.84	1.97	2.10	1.014	.37			
Group session 1	1.41	1.42	1.72	1.733	.19			
Group session 7	1.27	1.02	1.76	5.852	.005*	.10	.05	.01
Group session 11	1.16	.83	1.68	7.501	.001*		.01	.01
Group session 15	1.03	.80	1.51	4.225	.02*		.05	.01

				F	p			
HSCL-90 agitated depression factor								
Intake	1.61	1.85	1.79	.719	.49			
Individual session 1	1.39	1.54	1.60	.572	.57			
Group session 1	1.23	1.01	1.31	1.799	.17			
Group session 7	1.05	.72	1.33	5.529	.006*	.10	.10	.01
Group session 11	.89	.59	1.17	4.171	.02*	.05	.10	.01
Group session 15	.79	.55	1.13	4.987	.01*		.10	.01
Beck Depression Inventory								
Intake	26.77	28.13	31.85	3.106	.05*			
Individual session 1	25.56	25.70	26.95	.275	.76			
Group session 1	19.20	19.66	22.73	1.420	.25			
Group session 7	17.31	16.09	19.63	.832	.44			
Group session 11	14.76	12.99	20.89	4.802	.01*		.01	.01
Group session 15	11.11	10.78	20.86	8.451	.001*		.01	.01
Global Improvement Scale—Patient								
Individual session 1	3.68	3.94	4.17	1.002	.38			
Group session 1	4.56	4.22	4.47	.413	.66			
Group session 7	4.89	4.91	4.47	.758	.47			
Group session 11	5.12	4.76	4.69	2.562	.09			
Group session 15	5.02	5.29	4.79	3.185	.05*			

Note. CBT = cognitive-behavior therapy. IMI = imipramine. TRAD = traditional therapy.
*$P \leq .05$.

Table 3-8. End-point independent evaluator ratings on doctor's Hopkins Symptom Checklist 90 (HSCL-90—Dr.) clusters and Hamilton Rating Scale for Depression (HRSD)—total

	Means			F	P	Range test P		
	CBT alone	CBT + IMI	TRAD			CBT vs. CBT + IMI	CBT vs. TRAD	CBT + IMI vs. TRAD
HSCL-90—Dr. somatization								
Preevaluation	2.22	2.61	2.45	.425	.66			
Group session 1	2.38	1.96	2.58	2.044	.14			
Group session 7	2.18	1.86	2.43	1.521	.23			
Group session 11	2.31	1.43	2.28	3.571	.03*	.05		.05
Group session 15	2.16	1.27	2.03	4.086	.02*	.01		.05
HSCL-90—Dr. obsessive-compulsiveness								
Preevaluation	2.78	2.30	2.80	1.176	.32			
Group session 1	2.42	2.65	3.03	2.293	.11			
Group session 7	2.48	2.34	2.75	.714	.49			
Group session 11	2.34	1.85	2.56	1.968	.15			
Group session 15	2.31	1.93	2.72	2.468	.09			.05
HSCL-90—Dr. interpersonal sensitivity								
Preevaluation	3.26	2.61	3.20	2.318	.11			
Group session 1	3.07	3.05	2.99	.069	.93			
Group session 7	3.03	2.34	2.91	2.872	.06	.05		
Group session 11	2.73	2.58	2.84	.239	.79			
Group session 15	2.79	2.56	2.78	.405	.67			.10

				F	p			
HSCL-90 — Dr. depression								
Preevaluation	3.96	4.04	4.20	1.445	.24			
Group session 1	3.25	3.53	3.91	4.251	.02*		.01	.10
Group session 7	2.85	2.71	3.49	2.527	.09			
Group session 11	2.37	2.40	2.99	1.554	.22			
Group session 15	1.94	2.18	2.70	1.662	.20		.10	.05
HSCL-90 — Dr. anxiety								
Preevaluation	2.74	2.65	2.85	.161	.85			
Group session 1	2.85	2.37	3.02	2.506	.09			.05
Group session 7	2.52	2.10	2.93	3.249	.05*	.10		.01
Group session 11	2.26	2.05	2.85	2.421	.10			
Group session 15	2.23	1.99	2.96	4.086	.02*		.05	.01
HSCL-90 — Dr. anger-hostility								
Preevaluation	2.33	2.65	1.65	3.585	.03*			
Group session 1	2.27	2.08	2.45	.665	.52			
Group session 7	2.37	1.86	2.37	1.198	.31			
Group session 11	1.88	1.83	2.22	.657	.52			
Group session 15	2.03	1.79	1.99	.308	.74			
HSCL-90 — Dr. phobic anxiety								
Preevaluation	1.44	1.22	1.75	.861	.43			
Group session 1	1.34	.79	1.37	3.439	.04*	.05		.05
Group session 7	1.30	.11	1.30	16.578	.0001*	.01		.01
Group session 11	1.26	.30	1.14	7.896	.0001*	.01		.01
Group session 15	1.15	.37	.92	4.157	.02*	.01		.05

Table 3-8. End-point independent evaluator ratings on doctor's Hopkins Symptom Checklist 90 (HSCL-90−Dr.) clusters and Hamilton Rating Scale for Depression (HRSD)−total−Continued

	Means			F	P	Range test P		
	CBT alone	CBT + IMI	TRAD			CBT vs. CBT + IMI	CBT vs. TRAD	CBT + IMI vs. TRAD
HSCL-90−Dr. sleep								
Preevaluation	2.78	3.04	2.85	.235	.79			
Group session 1	2.35	2.05	2.91	2.990	.06	.10		.01
Group session 7	2.15	1.69	2.82	3.705	.03*	.10		.01
Group session 11	1.96	1.91	2.51	1.084	.34			
Group session 15	1.97	1.56	2.17	.962	.39			
HRSD								
Preevaluation	17.67	19.09	19.15	1.004	.37			
Group session 1	15.89	14.48	17.41	2.388	.10			.05
Group session 7	14.76	12.25	15.87	2.272	.11			
Group session 11	13.11	10.59	14.93	2.996	.06			.05
Group session 15	11.71	9.45	14.30	3.517	.04*		.10	.01

Note. CBT = cognitive-behavior therapy. IMI = imipramine. TRAD = traditional therapy.
*$P \leq .05$.

phase was made by the independent evaluator. This decision indicated that the initial treatment condition had failed to produce a meaningful reduction in depression, i.e., the patient still scored above the original entry criteria on patient and therapist ratings of depression, such as the BDI, the RDS, and the HRSD. In effect then, the percentage of patients within each treatment condition who were judged to require optimization serves as another index of treatment efficacy.

The clinical need for optimization was reliably greater for patients receiving traditional therapy (66.7%) than for patients receiving either CBT alone (17.4%) or CBT plus imipramine (27.8%; χ^2 = 9.02, df 2; P = .01). These data are consistent with other quantitative analyses that also supported the therapeutic advantage for the CBT conditions relative to traditional therapy. During optimization, only two of eight patients treated with traditional therapy showed improvement on the BDI, whereas two of four patients treated with CBT alone and four of five patients treated with CBT plus imipramine showed improvement. Of the eight patients who improved with optimization, one traditional therapy patient and one CBT plus imipramine patient showed complete remission of their depression, i.e., a BDI score of less than 10. The data after optimization were not used in the outcome analyses of the active phase.

Follow-up

Following the optimization phase in which 17 of the 53 patients who completed treatment were optimized, all patients were seen for monthly follow-up evaluations by their primary therapist and for quarterly blind evaluations by the independent evaluator.

Analyses of variance were done on Global Improvement Scale—Patient ratings at 3, 6, and 9 months. Borderline significance was found in favor of CBT alone and CBT plus imipramine in comparison with traditional therapy. Analyses of covariance with the initial-visit score (initial evaluation by independent evaluator) as the covariate were done with the BDI and the HRSD. BDI scores showed significant superiority of both CBT alone and CBT plus imipramine over traditional therapy at 3 and 9 months. HRSD scores showed significant differences in the same direction at 9 months. Newman-Keuls multiple range tests of differences between treatments showed a similar outcome pattern in patient and doctor ratings (Table 3-9).

Discussion

The CBT and CBT plus imipramine group patients improved significantly more in almost all areas of psychopathology than the traditional therapy group patients. We do not, however, feel confident

Table 3-9. Follow-up analyses

Scale	Month of follow-up	Mean CBT alone	n	CBT + IMI	n	TRAD	n	F	P	Neuman-Keuls P CBT vs. CBT + IMI	CBT vs. TRAD	CBT + IMI vs. TRAD
GIS-patient	3	5.84	19	5.43	15	4.86	7	2.458	.10			
	6	6.28	14	6.31	13	6.00	6	.332	.72			
	9	6.33	12	6.14	14	5.17	6	2.856	.07			
BDI	3	7.23	21	6.38	18	12.49	11	3.172	.05	NS	.05	.05
	6	8.78	19	4.83	16	10.56	7	2.05	.14			
	9	7.59	16	5.38	15	15.13	7	3.31	.05	NS	.05	.01
HRSD	3	7.32	23	6.07	18	8.33	11	.54	.59	NS		
	6	9.49	21	5.76	17	7.86	8	1.74				
	9	8.37	18	5.98	15	13.55	7	5.86	.01	NS	.05	.01

Note. CBT = cognitive-behavior therapy. IMI = imipramine. TRAD = traditional therapy. GIS = Global Improvement Scale. BDI = Beck Depression Inventory. HRSD = Hamilton Rating Scale for Depression.

in making a general statement about the efficacy of traditional group therapy in major depression because only one therapist was used and because, in actual practice, depressed patients are seldom treated in diagnostically homogeneous groups with this technique. Moreover, 15 group sessions over 12 weeks would not be considered an adequate period for a fair trial of this type of therapy. The main reason for use of the traditional group therapy was to provide a credible control for the influence of nonspecific group factors, such as cohesion, in the improvement of the CBT experimental subjects.

We found a trend, particularly in the independent evaluator ratings, for CBT plus imipramine to do better than CBT alone. The independent evaluator also tended to detect improvement earlier than the patients did in their self-ratings, a phenomenon well known to clinicians.

In the measures of social adjustment, CBT alone did significantly better than CBT plus imipramine, possibly reflecting an attribution effect: because patients on CBT alone could not rely on medication to improve depression, they may have tried harder to improve their relationship with others in order to overcome dysphoric feelings.

The finding of efficacy of CBT in this study confirms that of several other authors (Murphy et al. 1984; Roth et al. 1982), but differs from that of Jarvik et al. (1982), who found that geriatric depressive patients responded only weakly to group CBT and psychodynamic group therapy.

We compared our BDI scores before and after treatment with those of Rush et al. (1977) and Rush and Watkins (1981) and have the impression that group CBT in our hands was as effective as individual CBT in their studies. Although a direct comparison would be needed to confirm this impression, a comparison of BDI and HRSD scores of the studies by Rush and colleagues with our own results supports this impression (Tables 3-10 and 3-11).

It should be emphasized that the 61% complete remission rate that we observed in CBT-alone group patients after the active phase of treatment (i.e., 14 of 23 patients with BDI scores of 0–9) was almost exactly the mean improvement rate that was found by Rush (personal communication) in his survey of the results of CBT for depression studies. Operationally, this finding by Rush was based on the percentage of CBT "completer" patients who were reported to have posttreatment BDI scores in the nondepressed range of 0–9 in both published and ongoing studies.

With regard to the interaction of pharmacotherapy and psychotherapy, it must be noted that effects as measured by the HRSD seem to be stronger in combined CBT and imipramine. Also of interest is the effect on the anxiety factor of the HSCL-90, where CBT plus imipramine was superior to CBT alone. This finding is congruent with the findings of clinical psychopharmacological studies such as that by Kahn et al. (1986) where imipramine significantly reduced anxiety. Interestingly, this did not occur with the obsessive-compulsive factor, where only serotonergic antidepressants have proven effective (Perse 1988).

Because of the pilot nature of this study, several potential predictor variables were not examined. We are, however, presently conducting a larger study with additional control conditions. Patients are assigned to one of five experimental cells: 1) CBT, 2) CBT and placebo, 3) CBT and imipramine, 4) imipramine and clinical management, and 5) placebo and clinical management. In this study, a traditional group therapy control was omitted due to its poor performance in our earlier studies.

GENERAL CONCLUSIONS

The two studies reported herein indicate a low level of effectiveness for traditional free-interaction group psychotherapy with depressed patients if used without antidepressants. CBT, on the other hand, if conducted with a rigorous technique in closed groups, will obtain better results, although not as good as those seen when CBT is combined with antidepressants.

The effectiveness of CBT may be due more to the cognitive

Table 3-10. Comparison of Beck Depression Inventory scores for completers

	Hopkins[a]	Rush and Watkins 1981		Rush et al. 1977
	Group	Group	Individual	Individual
Pretreatment		29.2	29.5	30.28
(mean ± SD)	26.2 ± 5.5	6.2	7.8	6.82
	vs.			
Posttreatment				
(mean ± SD)	9.7 ± 8.1	16.2*	8.6	5.94
		12.8**	6.7	5.33
n	23	23	8	18

[a]Results are for patients treated at the Johns Hopkins Hospital Phipps Outpatient Department.
*9.7 vs. 16.2: $t = 2.10$, df 22; $P \leq .05$.
**8.1 vs. 12.8: $F = 2.50$, df 22,22; $P \leq .05$.

Table 3-11. Comparison of Hamilton Rating Scale for Depression scores for completers and completers plus deviators (end point)

	Hopkins[a] Completers		Rush et al. 1977 Individual completers		Hopkins[a] End point		Rush et al. 1977 Individual end point
Pretreatment (mean ± SD)	18.91 ± 4.5	vs.	21.20 ± 3.34		10.67 ± 4.6	vs.	20.94 ± 3.40
Posttreatment (mean ± SD)	10.11 ± 5.9		5.80* ± 3.67		11.20 ± 6.2		6.25 ± 3.98**
n	23		15		27		16

[a]Results are for patients treated at the Johns Hopkins Hospital Phipps Outpatient Department.
*t = 2.78, df 36; $P \leq$ .01.
**t = 3.91, df 41; $P \leq$ .005.

component than to the behavioral component of the therapy in view of the results of Roth et al. (1982). They used a behavior self-control technique in groups of depressive patients treated for 12 weeks. They also found that combining desipramine with behavior group therapy obtained superior results.

The combination of a benzodiazepine, such as diazepam, with group therapy did not result in a similar improvement in depressed outpatients. Although these results await confirmation by a replication now being completed, practical application in daily clinical practice confirms the generalization of these research findings (Covi and Primakoff 1988; Roth and Covi 1984).

Finally, follow-up studies confirm that the relative results of group traditional and cognitive therapies are maintained over a period of 9 months posttreatment.

REFERENCES

Barrett-Lenard GT: Dimension of therapist response as causal factors in therapeutic change. Psychological Monographs 76:1–36, 1962

Beck AT, Greenberg RL: Coping With Depression (booklet). New York, Institute for Rational Living, 1974

Beck AT, Ward DH, Mendelson M, et al: An inventory for measuring depression. Arch Gen Psychiatry 4:561–571, 1961

Beck AT, Rush AJ, Shaw BF, et al: Cognitive Therapy of Depression. New York, Guilford, 1979

Brotman AW, Folk WE, Gelenberg AJ: Pharmacological treatment of acute depressive subtypes, in Psychopharmacology, The Third Generation of Progress. Edited by Meltzer HY. New York, Raven, 1987, pp 1031–1040

Covi L, Lipman RS: Primary depression or primary anxiety? A possible psychometric approach to a diagnostic dilemma. Clinical Neuropsychopharmacology 7 (suppl 1): 924–925, 1984

Covi L, Lipman RS: Cognitive behavioral group psychotherapy combined with imipramine in major depression. Psychopharmacol Bull 23:173–176, 1987

Covi L, Primakoff L: Cognitive group therapy, in American Psychiatric Press Review of Psychiatry, Vol 7. Edited by Frances AJ, Hales RE. Washington, DC, American Psychiatric Press, 1988, pp 608–626

Covi L, Lipman RS, Derogatis LR, et al: Drugs and group psychotherapy in neurotic depression. Am J Psychiatry 131:191–198, 1974

Covi L, Lipman RS, Alarcon RD, et al: Drug and psychotherapy interactions in depression. Am J Psychiatry 133:502–508, 1976

Covi L, Lipman RS, McNair DM, et al: Symptomatic volunteers in multi-center drug trials. Prog Neuropsychopharmacol 3:521–533, 1980

Covi L, Roth D, Lipman RS: Cognitive group therapy of depression: the close-ended group. Am J Psychother 36:459–469, 1982

Covi L, Roth D, Pattison JH, et al: Group cognitive behavioral therapy of depression: two parallel manuals for a controlled study, in The Theory and Practice of Cognitive Therapy. Edited by Perris C, Perris H, Blackburn I. Heidelberg, Springer Verlag, 1988, pp 198–222

Derogatis LR, Lipman RS, Covi L: SCL-90: an outpatient psychiatric rating scale. Psychopharmacol Bull 9:13–25, 1973

Endicott J, Spitzer RL: A diagnostic interview: the Schedule for Affective Disorders and Schizophrenia. Arch Gen Psychiatry 35:837–844, 1978

Frank JD: Therapeutic components of psychotherapy: a 25 year progress report of research. J Nerv Ment Dis 159:325–342, 1974

Frank JD, Powdermaker FB: Group psychotherapy, in American Handbook of Psychiatry, Vol 2. Edited by Arieti S. New York, Basic Books, 1959, pp 1362–1374

Gardos G, DiMascio A, Salzman C, et al: Differential actions of chlordiazepoxide and oxazepam in hostility. Arch Gen Psychiatry 18:757–760, 1968

Guy W, Bonato RR: Manual for the ECDEU Assessment Battery, 2nd Revision. Chevy Chase, MD, National Institute of Mental Health, 1970

Hamilton MA: A rating scale for depression. J Neurol Neurosurg Psychiatry 23:56–62, 1960

Hoehn-Saric R, Frank J, Imber S, et al: Systematic preparation of patients for psychotherapy, I: effects on therapy behavior and outcome. J Psychiatry Res 2:267–281, 1964

Hollingshead AB: Two-Factor Index of Social Position. New Haven, CT, Yale University, 1957

Hollon SD, Shaw BF: Group cognitive therapy for depressed patients, in Cognitive Therapy for Depression. Edited by Beck AT, Rush AJ, Shaw BF, et al. New York, Guilford, 1979

Jarvik LF, Mintz J, Stener J, et al: Treating geriatric depression: a 26-week interim analysis. J Am Geriatr Soc 30:713–717, 1982

Jones M: Group treatment with particular reference to group projection methods. Am J Psychiatry 101:292–299, 1944

Kahn RJ, McNair DM, Lipman RS, et al: Imipramine and chlordiazepoxide in depressive and anxiety disorders, II: efficacy in anxious outpatients. Arch Gen Psychiatry 43:79–85, 1986

Kuhn R: The imipramine story, in Discoveries in Biological Psychiatry. Edited by Ayd FJ, Blackwell B. Philadelphia, PA, JB Lippincott, 1970

Lipman RS, Covi L: Outpatient treatment of neurotic depression: medication and group psychotherapy, in Evaluation of Psychological Therapies. Edited by Spitzer RL, Klein DF. Baltimore, MD, Johns Hopkins University Press, 1976

Lipman RS, Cole JO, Park LC, et al: Sensitivity of symptom and non-symptom-focused criteria of outpatient drug efficacy. Am J Psychiatry 122:24–27, 1965

Lipman RS, Covi L, Shapiro HK: The Hopkins Symptom Checklist (HSCL): factors derived from the HSCL-90. J Affective Disord 1:9–24, 1979

McNair DM, Lorr M: An analysis of mood in neurotics. J Abnorm Soc Psychol 69:620–627, 1964

Murphy GE, Simons AD, Wetzel RD, et al: Cognitive psychotherapy and pharmacotherapy. Arch Gen Psychiatry 41:33–41, 1984

Overall JR, Hollister LE, Johnson M, et al: Nosology of depression and differential response to drugs. JAMA 195:946–948, 1966

Perse T: Obsessive compulsive disorders: a treatment review. J Clin Psychiatry 49:48–85, 1988

Primakoff L, Epstein N, Covi L: Homework compliance: an uncontrolled variable in cognitive therapy outcome research. Behavior Therapy 17:433–446, 1986

Raskin A: The prediction of antidepressant drug effects: review and critique, in Psychopl.armacology: A Review of Progress, 1957–1967. Edited by Efron DH. Washington, DC, U.S. Government Printing Office, 1968, pp 757–765

Raskin A, Schulterrbrandt JG, Boothe H, et al: Treatment, social and psychiatric history variables related to symptom reduction in hospitalized depressions, in Psychopharmacology and the Individual Patient. Edited by Wittenborn JR, Goldberg SC, May PRA. New York, Raven, 1970, pp 135–159

Roth D, Covi L: Cognitive group psychotherapy of depression: the open-ended group. Int J Group Psychother 34:67–82, 1984

Roth D, Bielski R, Jones M, et al: A comparison of self-control therapy and combined self-control therapy and antidepressant medication in the treatment of depression. Behavior Therapy 13:133–144, 1982

Rush AJ, Watkins JT: Group versus individual cognitive therapy: a pilot study. Cognitive Therapy Research 5:95–103, 1981

Rush AJ, Beck AT, Kovacs M, et al: Comparative efficacy of cognitive therapy and pharmacotherapy in the treatment of depressed patients. Cognitive Therapy Research 1:17–37, 1977

Slavson SR: Criteria for selection and rejection of patients for various types of group psychotherapy. Int J Group Psychother 5:3–30, 1955

Spitzer RL, Endicott J, Robins E: Research Diagnostic Criteria (RDC) for a Selected Group of Functional Disorders, 3rd Edition. New York, Biometrics Research, 1978

Uhlenhuth EH, Lipman RS, Covi L: Combined pharmacotherapy and psychotherapy. J Nerv Ment Dis 148:52–64, 1969

Weissman AN: The dysfunctional attitude scale: a validation study. Dissertation Abstracts International 40:1389b–1390b, 1979

Weissman MM, Bothwell S: Assessment of social adjustment by patient self-report. Arch Gen Psychiatry 33:1111–1115, 1976

Williams HV, Lipman RS, Rickels K: Replications of symptom distress factors in anxious neurotic outpatients. Multivariate Behavior Research 3:199–213, 1968

Wolf A: Group psychotherapy, in Comprehensive Textbook of Psychiatry, 1st Edition. Edited by Freedman AM, Kaplan HJ, Kaplan HS. Baltimore, MD, Williams & Wilkins, 1967, pp 1234–1241

Yalom ID: The Theory and Practice of Group Psychotherapy, 1st Edition. New York, Basic Books, 1970

Chapter 4

Interpersonal Psychotherapy and Its Derivatives in the Treatment of Depression

Myrna M. Weissman, Ph.D.
Gerald L. Klerman, M.D.

Chapter 4

Interpersonal Psychotherapy and Its Derivatives in the Treatment of Depression

Interpersonal psychotherapy (IPT) is based on the evidence that most clinical depressions—regardless of symptom patterns, severity, biological vulnerability, or personality traits—occur in an interpersonal context. Understanding and renegotiating the interpersonal context associated with the depression can aid in the depressed person's recovery and reduce social morbidity.

IPT is a brief (usually 12–16 weeks), weekly psychotherapeutic treatment developed for the ambulatory, nonbipolar, nonpsychotic, depressed patient, focused on improving the quality of the depressed patient's current interpersonal functioning and identifying the problems associated with the onset of depression. It is suitable for use, after appropriate training, by experienced psychiatrists, psychologists, and social workers. It can be used alone or with pharmacologic approaches.

IPT has evolved from over 20 years of experience in the treatment and research of ambulatory depressed patients. It has been tested alone and in comparison and in combination with tricyclics in six clinical trials with depressed patients —three of maintenance (Klerman et al. 1974; Frank et al. 1989; Reynold and Imber 1988) and three of acute (Elkin et al. 1986; Sloane et al. 1985; Weissman et al. 1979) treatment. Two derivative forms of IPT, conjoint marital (Foley et al. 1990) and interpersonal counseling (Klerman et al. 1987), have been developed and tested in pilot studies. Six studies have included a drug comparison group (Elkin et al. 1986; Klerman et al. 1974; Frank et al. 1989; Reynold and Imber 1988; Sloane et al. 1985; Weissman et al. 1979), and four have included a combination of IPT and drugs (Elkin et al. 1986; Klerman et al. 1974; Sloane et al. 1985; Weissman et al. 1979).

The concept, techniques, and methods of IPT have been operationally described in a manual that has undergone a number of revisions. This manual, now in book form (Klerman et al. 1984), was developed to standardize the treatment so that clinical trials could be undertaken. A training program for experienced psychotherapists of different disciplines providing the treatment for these clinical trials has been developed (Weissman et al. 1982). There is to our knowledge no ongoing training program for practitioners, although workshops are available from time to time, and the book can serve as a guide for the experienced clinician who wants to learn IPT.

It is our experience that various treatments may be suitable for depression and that the depressed patient's interests are best served by the availability and scientific testing of different psychological, as well as pharmacological, treatments, to be used alone or in combination. Ultimately, clinical testing and experience will determine which is the best treatment for the particular patient. This chapter describes the theoretical and empirical basis for IPT, the efficacy studies with ambulatory depressed patients, and the two new derivative forms of IPT.

THEORETICAL AND EMPIRICAL BACKGROUND

Our treatment and research activities derive from numerous theoretical and empirical sources.

Theoretical Sources

The ideas of Adolf Meyer, whose prominent psychobiological approach to understanding psychiatric disorders placed great emphasis on the patient's environment, comprise the most prominent theoretical sources for IPT (Meyer 1957). Meyer viewed psychiatric disorders as an expression of the patient's attempt to adapt to his or her environment. An individual's response to environmental change is determined by prior experiences, particularly early experiences in the family and the individual's affiliation with various social groups. Among Meyer's associates, Harry Stack Sullivan stands out for his general theory of interpersonal relationships and for his writings linking clinical psychiatry to the emerging social sciences (Sullivan 1953).

Empirical Sources

The empirical basis for understanding and treating depression with IPT includes studies associating stress and life events with the onset of depression; longitudinal studies demonstrating the social impairment of depressed women during the acute depressive phase and the following symptomatic recovery; studies by Brown et al. (1977) that demonstrate the role of intimacy and social supports as protection against depression in the face of adverse life stress; and studies by Pearlin and Lieberman (1979) and Ilfield (1977) that show the impact of chronic social and interpersonal stress, particularly marital stress, on the onset of depression. The works of Bowlby (1969) and Henderson et al. (1978) emphasize the importance of attachment bonds or, conversely, show that the loss of social attachments can be associated with the onset of depression, and finally, recent epidemiologic data show a strong association between marital disputes and major depression (Weissman 1987).

CHARACTERISTICS OF IPT

Nature of Changes in Depression With IPT

Depression may be seen as involving three components:

1. *Symptom formation,* involving the development of the depressive affect and vegetative signs and symptoms, which may derive from psychobiological and/or psychodynamic mechanisms.
2. Social functioning, involving social interactions with other persons, which derive from learning based on childhood experiences, concurrent social reinforcement, and/or current personal mastery and competence.
3. Personality, involving more enduring traits and behaviors—the handling of anger and guilt and overall self-esteem—that constitute the person's unique reactions and patterns of functioning and that also may contribute to a predisposition to manifest symptom episodes.

IPT attempts to intervene in the first two processes. Because of the brevity of the treatment, the low level of psychotherapeutic intensity, and the focus on the context of the current depressive episode, no claim is made that IPT will have an impact on the enduring aspects of personality, although personality functioning is assessed.

Goals of IPT for Depression

IPT develops directly from an interpersonal conceptualization of depression. IPT does not, however, assume that interpersonal problems "cause" depression, but, rather, that whatever the cause, depression occurs in an interpersonal context. The therapeutic strategies of IPT are to understand that context and to resolve the dispute. As noted before, IPT is not expected to have a marked impact on enduring aspects of personality structure. Although some longer-term psychotherapies have been designed to achieve personality change by use of the interpersonal approach (Arietti and Bemporad 1979), these treatments have not been assessed in controlled trials.

IPT facilitates recovery from acute depression by relieving depressive symptoms and by helping the patient become more effective in dealing with current interpersonal problems that are associated with the onset of symptoms. Symptom relief begins with helping the patient understand that the vague and uncomfortable symptoms are part of a known syndrome, which is well described, understood, and relatively common, and which responds to various treatments and has good prognosis. Psychopharmacologic approaches may be used in conjunction with IPT to alleviate symptoms more rapidly. Table 4-1 describes the stages and tasks in the conduct of IPT.

Table 4-1.   Stages and tasks in the conduct of interpersonal psychotherapy

Stages	Tasks
Early	• **Treatment of depressive symptoms** Review of symptoms Confirmation of diagnosis Communication of diagnosis to patient Evaluation of medication need Education of patient about depression (epidemiology, symptoms, clinical course, treatment prognosis) Legitimation of patient's "sick role" • **Assessment of interpersonal relations** Inventory of current relationships Choice of interpersonal problem area • **Therapeutic contract** Statement of goals, diagnosis, problem areas Medication plan Agreement
Middle	• **Treatment focusing on problem area** Unresolved grief Interpersonal disputes Role transition Interpersonal deficits
Termination	

Treating the depressed patient's problems in interpersonal relations begins with exploring which of four problem areas commonly associated with the onset of depression—grief, role disputes, role transition, or interpersonal deficit—is related to the patient's depression. IPT then focuses on the particular interpersonal problem as it relates to the onset of depression (Klerman et al. 1987).

IPT Compared With Other Psychotherapies

The procedures and techniques of many psychotherapies have much in common. Many therapies emphasize helping the patient develop a sense of mastery, combat social isolation, restore the patient's feeling of group belonging, and help the patient rediscover meaning in life. The psychotherapies differ, however, as to whether the patient's problems lie in the far past, the immediate past, or the present. IPT focuses primarily on the patient's present, and it differs from other psychotherapies in its limited duration, its attention to current depressive symptoms, and the current depression-related interpersonal context. Given this frame of reference, IPT includes a systematic review of the patient's current relations with significant others.

IPT is time limited and not long-term. Considerable research has demonstrated the value of short-term, time-limited psychotherapies (usually once a week for less than 9–12 months) for many depressed outpatients (Klerman et al. 1987). Although long-term treatment may still be required for chronic personality disorders, particularly maladaptive interpersonal and cognitive patterns, and for ameliorating or replacing dysfunctional social skills, evidence for the efficacy of long-term psychotherapy is limited. Long-term treatment also has the potential disadvantage of promoting dependence and reinforcing avoidance behavior. Psychotherapies that are short-term or time limited aim to minimize these adverse effects.

IPT is focused and not open-ended. In common with other brief psychotherapies, IPT focuses on one or two problem areas in the patient's current interpersonal functioning, and the focus is agreed on by the patient and the psychotherapist after initial evaluation sessions. The topical content of sessions is, therefore, focused and not open-ended.

IPT deals with current, not past, interpersonal relationships, focusing on the patient's immediate social context just before and as it has been since the onset of the current depressive episode. Past depressive episodes, early family relationships, and previous significant relationships and friendship patterns are assessed, however, in order to understand overall patterns in the patient's interpersonal relationships.

IPT is concerned with interpersonal, not intrapsychic, phenomena.

In exploring current interpersonal problems with the patient, the psychotherapist may observe the operation of intrapsychic mechanisms such as projection, denial, isolation, or repression. In IPT, however, the psychotherapist does not work on helping the patient see the current situation as a manifestation of internal conflict but rather explores the patient's current psychiatric behavior in terms of interpersonal relations.

EFFICACY OF IPT

A major effort in our work has been testing the efficacy of treatment by the application of the techniques of the randomized clinical trials designed to assess pharmacotherapy, psychotherapy, and the combination of both. Table 4-2 describes the efficacy of IPT and its derivatives (see Weissman et al. 1987 for complete description).

IPT as Maintenance Treatment

The first study of IPT began in 1967 and investigated maintenance treatment (Klerman et al. 1974; see Table 4-2). In June 1967, it was clear that the tricyclic antidepressants were efficacious in the treatment of acute depression. It was unclear how long treatment should continue and what the role of psychotherapy was in maintenance treatment. Our study was designed to answer those questions.

We studied 150 acutely depressed outpatients who had responded to a tricyclic antidepressant (amitriptyline) with symptom reduction. Each patient received 8 months of maintenance treatment with drugs alone, psychotherapy (IPT) alone, or a combination of both. We found that maintenance drug treatment prevented relapse and that psychotherapy alone improved social functioning and interpersonal relations, but had no effect on symptomatic relapse. Because of the differential effects of the treatments, the combination of drugs and psychotherapy was the most efficacious (Klerman et al. 1974), and no negative interactions between drugs and psychotherapy were found.

In the course of that project, we became aware of the need for greater specification of the psychotherapeutic techniques involved and for the careful training of psychotherapists for research. The psychotherapy had been described in terms of conceptual framework, goals, frequency of contacts, and criteria for therapist suitability. However, the techniques and strategies and actual procedures had not been set out in a procedures manual, and there were no training programs available.

IPT as Acute Treatment

In 1973, we initiated a 16-week study of the acute treatment of 81

Table 4-2. Efficacy studies of interpersonal psychotherapy (IPT) and its derivatives

Reference	Treatment condition	Diagnosis (no patients)	Time (weeks)
Acute treatment studies			
Weissman et al. 1979	IPT + amitriptyline/amitriptyline/IPT/nonscheduled treatment	MDD ($N = 96$)	16
Sloane et al. 1985	IPT/nortriptyline/placebo	MDD or dysthymia, ages 60+ ($N = 30$)	6
Elkin et al. 1986	IPT/CB/imipramine + management/placebo + management	MDD ($N = 250$)	16
Maintenance treatment studies			
Klerman et al. 1974	IPT/low contact + amitriptyline/placebo/no pill	Recovered MDD ($N = 150$)	32
Frank et al. 1989	IPT/IPT + placebo/IPT + imipramine/ management + imipramine/management + placebo	Recovered recurrent MDD ($N = 125$)	3 years
Reynold and Imber 1988	Same design as Frank et al. 1989	Recovered recurrent MDD geriatric ($N = 120$)	3 years
Derivative IPT			
Foley et al. 1990	IPT-CM vs. individual IPT for marital disputes	MDD + marital disputes ($N = 18$)	16
Klerman et al. 1987	Interpersonal counseling for distress (IPC)	High-score GHQ ($N = 64$)	6

Note. MDD = major depressive disorder. CB = cognitive therapy. IPT-CM = conjoint marital interpersonal psychotherapy. GHQ = General Health Questionnaire.

ambulatory depressed patients, both men and women, using IPT and amitriptyline, each alone and in combination, against a nonscheduled psychotherapy treatment (DiMascio et al. 1979; Weissman et al. 1979; Table 4-2). IPT was administered weekly by experienced psychiatrists. A much more specific procedures manual for IPT was developed. By 1973, the Schedule for Affective Disorders and Schizophrenia (SADS) Research Diagnostic Criteria (RDC) were available for making more precise diagnostic judgments, thereby ensuring the selection of a more homogeneous sample of depressed patients (Endicott and Spitzer 1978).

Patients were assigned randomly to IPT or the control treatment at the beginning of treatment, which was limited to 16 weeks because this was an acute and not a maintenance treatment trial (Weissman et al. 1981). Patients were assessed up to 1 year after treatment had ended to determine any long-term treatment effects. The assessment of outcome was made by a clinical evaluator, who was independent of and blind to the treatment the patient was receiving.

In the latter part of the 1970s, we reported the results of IPT compared with tricyclic antidepressant treatment alone and their combination for acute depressions. We demonstrated that both active treatments, IPT and the tricylic, were more effective than the control treatment and that combined treatment was superior to either treatment (DiMascio et al. 1979; Weissman et al. 1979).

In addition, we conducted a 1-year follow-up study that indicated that the therapeutic benefit of treatment was sustained for most patients. Patients who had received IPT either alone or in combination with drugs were functioning better than patients who had received either drugs alone or the control treatment (Weissman et al. 1981). There remains a fraction of patients in all treatments who relapsed and for whom additional treatment was required.

Other Studies of IPT for Depression

Other researchers have now extended IPT to other aspects of depression. A long-term maintenance period of IPT is still underway at the University of Pittsburgh to assess the value of drugs and psychotherapy in maintenance treatment of chronic recurrent depressions (Frank et al. 1989; Table 4-2). A similar study in a depressed geriatric patient population is also underway at the University of Pittsburgh (Reynold and Imber 1988; Table 4-2). Also, Sloane et al. (1985; Table 4-2) completed a 6-week pilot trial of IPT compared with nortriptyline and placebo for depressed elderly patients. They found partial evidence that the efficacy of IPT over nortriptyline for elderly patients was due to the elderly not tolerating the medication.

The problem of medication in the elderly, particularly the anticholinergic effect, has led to the interest in psychotherapy in this age-group.

National Institute of Mental Health (NIMH) Collaborative Study of the Treatment of Depression

In the late 1970s, having efficacy data on two specified psychotherapies for ambulatory depressive patients, the NIMH, under the leadership of Drs. Parloff and Elkin, designed and initiated a multicenter, controlled, clinical trial of drugs and psychotherapy in the treatment of depression (Elkin et al. 1986; Table 4-2). Two hundred fifty outpatients were randomly assigned to four treatment conditions: 1) cognitive therapy, 2) IPT, 3) imipramine, or 4) a placebo–clinical management combination. Each patient was treated for 16 weeks. Extensive efforts were made in the selection and training of psychotherapists. Outcome was assessed by a battery of scales that assessed symptoms, social functioning, and cognition. The initial entry criterion was a score of at least 14 on the 17-item Hamilton Rating Scale for Depression (HRSD; Hamilton 1960). Of the 250 patients who entered treatment, 68% completed at least 15 weeks and 12 sessions of treatment. The preliminary findings from three centers (Oklahoma City; Washington, DC; Pittsburgh) were reported at the American Psychiatric Association annual meeting, 13 May 1986, in Washington, DC (Elkin et al. 1986). The full data have not yet been published. Overall, the findings showed that all active treatments were superior to placebo in the reduction of symptoms over a 16-week period. Other findings included

1. The overall degree of improvement was highly significant clinically. Over two-thirds of the patients were symptom free at the end of treatment.
2. More patients in the placebo–clinical management condition dropped out or were withdrawn, twice as many as for IPT, which had the lowest attrition rate.
3. At the end of 12 weeks of treatment, the two psychotherapies and imipramine were equivalent in the reduction of depressive symptoms and in overall functioning.
4. The pharmacotherapy (imipramine) had rapid initial onset of action, but by 12 weeks, the two psychotherapies had produced equivalent results.
5. Although many of the patients who were less severely depressed at intake improved with all treatment conditions, including the

placebo group, more severely depressed patients in the placebo group did poorly.

6. For the less severely depressed group, there were no differences among the treatments.

7. Forty-four percent of the sample was severely depressed at intake. The criteria of severity used was a score of 20 or more on the HRSD at entrance into the study. Patients in the IPT and the imipramine groups consistently and significantly had better scores than the placebo group on the HRSD. Only one of the psychotherapies, IPT, was significantly superior to placebo for the severely depressed group. For the severely depressed patients, IPT did as well as imipramine.

8. Surprisingly, one of the more important predictors of patient response to IPT was the presence of an endogenous depressive symptom picture measured by RDC after an interview with the SADS. This was also true for imipramine; however, this finding for drugs would have been expected from previous research.

DERIVATIVES OF IPT

IPT in a Conjoint Marital Context

Although the causal direction is unknown, clinical and epidemiologic studies have shown that marital disputes, separation, and divorce are strongly associated with the onset of depression (Weissman 1987). Moreover, depressed patients in ambulatory treatment frequently present marital problems as their chief complaint (Rounsaville et al. 1979, 1980). Yet, when psychotherapy is prescribed, it is unclear whether the patient, the couple, or the entire family should be involved. Some evidence suggests that individual psychotherapy for depressed patients involved in marital disputes may promote premature separation or divorce (Gurman and Kniskern 1978; Locke and Wallace 1976). There have been no published clinical trials comparing the efficacy of individual versus conjoint psychotherapy for depressed patients with marital problems.

We found that marital disputes often remained a complaint of the depressed patient despite the patient's symptomatic improvement with drugs or psychotherapy (Rounsaville et al. 1980). Because IPT presents strategies for managing the social and interpersonal problems associated with the onset of depressive symptoms, we speculated that a conjoint version of IPT, which focused intensively on problems in the marital relationship, would be useful in alleviating those problems (Foley et al. 1990; Table 4-2).

Individual IPT was adapted to the treatment of depression in the context of marital disputes by concentrating its focus on a subset of one of four problem areas associated with depression for which IPT was developed—interpersonal marriage disputes. IPT–conjoint marital (IPT-CM) extends individual IPT techniques for use with the identified patient and his or her spouse. The treatment incorporates aspects of currently available marital therapies, particularly those that emphasize dysfunctional communication as the focus of interventions. In IPT-CM, functioning of the couple is assessed in five general areas: communication, intimacy, boundary management, leadership, and attainment of socially appropriate goals. Dysfunctional behavior in these areas is noted, and treatment is focused on bringing about improvement in a small number of target problem areas. A treatment manual and a training program like those used in IPT were developed for IPT-CM in the initial phase of this study.

Only patients who identified marital disputes as the major problem associated with the onset or exacerbation of a major depression were admitted into a pilot study. Patients were randomly assigned to IPT or IPT-CM and received 16 weekly therapy sessions. In IPT-CM, the spouse was required to participate in all psychotherapy sessions, whereas in IPT the spouse did not meet with the therapist. Patients and spouses in both treatment conditions were asked to refrain from taking psychotropic medication during the study without first discussing it with their therapists; therapists were discouraged from prescribing or arranging for prescriptions of any psychotropic medication.

Three therapists (a psychiatrist, a psychologist, and a social worker) administered individual IPT to depressed married subjects. Three therapists (social workers) administered IPT-CM. All therapists had extensive prior experience in the treatment of depressed patients. At the end of treatment, patients in both groups expressed satisfaction with the treatment, felt that they had improved, and attributed improvement to their therapy (Table 4-3). Patients in both groups exhibited a significant reduction in symptoms of depression and social impairment from intake to termination of therapy. There was no significant difference between treatment groups in the degree of improvement in depressive symptoms and social functioning by end point (Foley et al. 1990).

Locke-Wallace Marital Adjustment Test (Locke and Wallace 1976) scores at session 16 were significantly higher (indicative of better marital adjustment) for patients receiving IPT-CM than for patients receiving IPT. Scores on the Spanier Dyadic Adjustment Scale (Spanier 1976) also indicated greater improvement in marital functioning for patients receiving IPT-CM than for patients receiving IPT. At session 16, patients receiving IPT-CM reported significantly higher levels of improvement in affectional expression (i.e., demonstrations of affection and sexual relations in the marriage) than patients receiving IPT.

The results should be interpreted with caution due to the pilot nature of the study—the small size of the pilot sample, the lack of a no-treatment control group, and the absence of a pharmacotherapy or a combined pharmacotherapy-psychotherapy comparison group. If the study were repeated, we would recommend that medication be freely allowed or used as a comparison condition and that there be more effort to reduce the symptom depression before proceeding to undertake the marital issue.

Interpersonal Counseling for Stress or Distress

Previous investigations have documented high frequencies of anxiety, depression, and functional bodily complaints in patients in primary-care settings (Brodaty and Andrews 1983; Goldberg 1972; Hoeper et al. 1979). Although some of these patients have diagnosable psychiatric disorders, a large percentage have symptoms that do not meet established criteria for psychiatric disorders. A mental health research program formed in a large health maintenance organization in the greater Boston area found that "problems of living" and symptoms of anxiety and depression were among the main reasons for individual primary-care visits. These clinical problems contribute heavily to high utilization of ambulatory services.

Table 4-3.   Symptom and social functioning scores at end of treatment in depressed patients with marital disputes receiving interpersonal psychotherapy (IPT) versus IPT in a conjoint marital context (IPT-CM)

	Treatment condition	
Outcomes at termination	IPT (n = 9)	IPT-CM (n = 9)
Depressive symptoms (Hamilton Rating Scale for Depression)	12.4	13.0
Overall social functioning	2.8	3.0
Marital adjustment (Locke-Wallace)[a]	4.7	5.8**
Affectional expression (Spanier Dyadic)[a]	6.5	8.6*

[a]Higher score indicates better marital adjustment.
*$P < .10$. **$P < .05$.

We developed a brief psychosocial intervention, interpersonal counseling (IPC), to deal with patients' symptoms of distress. IPC is a brief, focused, psychosocial intervention for administration by nurse practitioners working in a primary-care setting (Weissman and Klerman 1988). It was modified from IPT over a 6-month period, through an interactive and iterative process in which the research team met on a weekly basis with the nurse practitioners to review previous clinical experience, discuss case examples, observe videotapes, and listen to tape recordings.

IPC comprises a maximum of six half-hour counseling sessions in the primary-care office, focused on the patient's current functioning. Particular attention is given to recent changes in life events; sources of stress in the family, home, and workplace; friendship patterns; and ongoing difficulties in interpersonal relations. IPC assumes that such events provide the interpersonal context in which bodily and emotional symptoms related to anxiety, depression, and distress occur. The treatment manual includes session-by-session instructions as to the purpose and methods for IPC, including "scripts" to ensure comparability of procedures among the nurse counselors.

Subjects with scores of 6 or higher were selected for assignment to an experimental group that offered IPC or to a comparison group that was followed naturalistically (Klerman et al. 1987; Table 4-2). Subjects selected for IPC were contacted by telephone and invited to make a prompt appointment with one of the study's nurse practitioners. During this telephone contact, reference was made to items of concern raised by the patient's response to the General Health Questionnaire (GHQ; Goldberg 1972), and the patient was offered an appointment to address these and other health issues of concern. Sixty-four patients were compared with a subgroup of 64 sex-matched untreated subjects with similar elevations in GHQ scores during June 1984.

IPC proved feasible in the primary-care environment (Klerman et al. 1987). It was easily learned by experienced nurse practitioners in a short (8–12 hours) training program. The brevity of the sessions and short duration of treatment rendered IPC compatible with usual professional practices in a primary-care unit. No significant negative effects of treatment were observed, and nurses were able with weekly supervision to counsel several patients whose levels of psychiatric distress would normally have resulted in direct referral to specialty mental health care. Compared with a group of untreated subjects with initial elevations in GHQ scores, patients receiving the IPC intervention showed greater reduction in symptom scores over an average interval of 3 months. Many IPC-treated patients reported relief of symptoms after only 1 or 2 sessions. Many of the patients met the criteria for depression when they entered the study.

This pilot study provides preliminary evidence that early detection and outreach to distressed adults, followed by brief treatment with IPC, can, in the short term, reduce symptoms of distress as measured by the GHQ. The main effect seems to occur in symptoms related to mood, especially in those forms of mild and moderate depression that are commonly seen in medical patients. Such outreach to distressed individuals may also result in reduction in utilization of health care services and avoidance of the need for medication.

Although definitive evaluation of IPC awaits further study and its effect on utilization is not yet determined, this report of short-term symptom reduction suggests that this approach to outreach and early intervention is an effective alternative to current practices. If so, then IPC may be a useful addition to the repertoire of psychosocial intervention skills that can be incorporated into routine primary care.

CONCLUSION

Current Role of IPT in the Psychotherapy of Depression

Although the positive findings of the clinical trials of IPT in the NIMH Collaborative Study and the other studies described are encouraging and have received considerable attention in the popular press (see Boffey 1986), we emphasize a number of limitations in the possible conclusion regarding the place of psychotherapy in the treatment of depression. All the studies, including those by our group and by the NIMH, were conducted on ambulatory depressed patients or patients experiencing distress. There are no systematic studies evaluating the efficacy of psychotherapy for hospitalized depressed patients or bipolar patients, who are usually more severely disabled and often suicidal.

It is also important to recognize that these results should not be interpreted as implying that all forms of psychotherapy are effective for depression. One significant feature of recent advances in psychotherapy research is in the development of psychotherapies specifically designed for depression—time-limited and of brief duration. Just as there are specific forms of medication, there are specific forms of psychotherapy. It would be an error to conclude that all forms of medication are useful for all types of depression; so it would be an error to conclude that all forms of psychotherapy are efficacious for all forms of depression.

These investigations indicate that for outpatient ambulatory depressed patients, there is a range of effective treatments, including a number of forms of brief psychotherapy and various medications, notably monoamine oxidase inhibitors and tricyclic antidepressants. These therapeutic advances have contributed to our understanding of the complex interplay of psychosocial and biological factors in the etiology and pathogenesis of depression, particularly ambulatory depression.

IPT and Pharmacotherapy Combined

Numerous studies described above compared IPT with medication and also evaluated the combination of IPT plus medication. Unlike other forms of psychotherapy, we have no ideological hesitation in prescribing medication. The decision to use medication in the treatment of depression should be based on the patient's severity of symptoms, quality of depression, duration of disability, and response to previous treatments. It should not be based on the loyalties or training of the professional, as is too often the case in common clinical practice.

In our studies, IPT and medication, usually tricyclic antidepressants, have had independent additive effects; on some measures, there have been suggestions of synergistic effects. We have found no negative interactions, and, in fact, patients treated with the combination of medication and psychotherapy have a lower dropout rate, a greater acceptance of the treatment program, and more rapid and pervasive symptom improvement. Contrary to many theoretical discussions, the prescription of medication does not interfere with the patient's capacity to participate in psychotherapy. In fact, the opposite occurs: a reduced discussion of symptoms facilitates the patient's capacity to make use of social learning.

Various treatments may be suitable for depression. The depressed patient's interests are best served by the availability and scientific testing of different psychological and pharmacological treatments, which can be used alone or in combination. The ultimate aim of these studies is to determine which treatments are best for specific subgroups of depressed patients.

REFERENCES

Arietti S, Bemporad J: Severe-Mild Depression: The Psychotherapeutic Approach. New York, Basic Books, 1979

Boffey PM: Psychotherapy is as good as drug in curing depression, study finds. New York Times, May 14, 1986, pp A1, A17

Bowlby J: Attachment and Loss, Vol 1. London, Hogarth Press, 1969

Brodaty H, Andrews G: Brief psychotherapy in family practice: a controlled perspective intervention trial. Br J Psychiatry 143:11–19, 1983

Brown GW, Harris T, Copeland JR: Depression and loss. Br J Psychiatry 130:1–18, 1977

DiMascio A, Weissman MM, Prusoff BA, et al: Differential symptom reduction by drugs and psychotherapy in acute depression. Arch Gen Psychiatry 36:1450–1456, 1979

Elkin I, Watkins R, Docherty J, et al: The NIMH Collaborative Program on the treatment of outpatient depression: preliminary results. Paper presented at the American Psychiatric Association annual meeting, Chicago, IL, May 1986

Endicott J, Spitzer RL: A diagnostic interview: the Schedule for Affective Disorders and Schizophrenia. Arch Gen Psychiatry 35:773–782, 1978

Foley SH, Rounsaville BJ, Weissman MM, et al: Individual versus conjoint interpersonal psychotherapy for depressed patients with marital disputes. International Journal of Family Psychiatry (in press)

Frank E, Kupfer D, Perel J: Early recurrence in unipolar depression. Arch Gen Psychiatry 46:397–400, 1989

Goldberg DP: The detection of psychiatric illness by questionnaire (Institute of Psychiatry, Maudsley Monographs No 21). London, Oxford University Press, 1972

Gurman AS, Kniskern DP: Research on marital and family therapy: progress, perspective and prospect, in Handbook of Psychotherapy and Behavior Change. Edited by Garfield S, Bergin A. New York, John Wiley, 1978, pp 817–902

Hamilton M: A rating scale for depression. J Neurol Neurosurg Psychiatry 23:56–62, 1960

Henderson S, Byrne DG, Duncan-Jones P, et al: Social bonds in the epidemiology of neurosis. Br J Psychiatry 132:463–466, 1978

Hoeper EW, Nycz GR, Cleary PH, et al: Estimated prevalence of RDC mental disorder in primary medical care. International Journal of Mental Health 8:6–15, 1979

Ilfield FW: Current social stressors and symptoms of depression. Am J Psychiatry 134:161–166, 1977

Klerman GL, DiMascio A, Weissman MM, et al: Treatment of depression by drugs and psychotherapy. Am J Psychiatry 131:186–191, 1974

Klerman GL, Weissman MM, Rounsaville BJ, et al: Interpersonal Psychotherapy of Depression. New York, Basic Books, 1984

Klerman GL, Budman S, Berwick D, et al: Efficacy of a brief psychosocial intervention for symptoms of stress and distress among patients in primary care. Med Care 25:1078–1088, 1987

Locke HJ, Wallace KM: Short-term marital adjustment and prediction tests: their reliability and validity. Marriage and Family Living 38:15–25, 1976

Meyer A: Psychobiology: A Science of Man. Springfield, IL, Charles C Thomas, 1957

Pearlin LI, Lieberman MA: Social sources of emotional distress, in Research in Community and Mental Health, Vol 1. Edited by Simmons R. Greenwich, CT, JAI, 1979, pp 217–248

Reynold C, Imber S: Unpublished manuscript. Pittsburgh, PA, University of Pittsburgh, 1988

Rounsaville BJ, Weissman MM, Prusoff BA, et al: Marital disputes and treatment outcome in depressed women. Compr Psychiatry 20:483–490, 1979

Rounsaville BJ, Prusoff BA, Weissman MM: The course of marital disputes in depressed women: a 48 month follow-up study. Compr Psychiatry 21:111–118, 1980

Sloane RB, Staples FR, Schneider LS: Interpersonal therapy versus nortrip-tyline for depression in the elderly, in Clinical and Pharmacological Studies in Psychiatric Disorders (Biographical Psychiatry—New Prospects No 5). Edited by Burrows GD, Norman TR, Dennerstein L. London, John Libbey, 1985, pp 344–346

Spanier GB: Measuring dyadic adjustment: new scales for assessing the quality of marriage and similar dyads. Journal of Marriage and Family Living 38:15–25, 1976

Sullivan HS: The Interpersonal Theory of Psychiatry. New York, WW Norton, 1953

Weissman MM: Advances in psychiatric epidemiology: rates and risks for major depression. Am J Public Health 77:445–451, 1987

Weissman MM, Klerman GL: Manual for interpersonal counseling for stress and distress. Unpublished manuscript, 1988

Weissman MM, Prusoff BA, DiMascio A, et al: The efficacy of drugs and psychotherapy in the treatment of acute depressive episodes. Am J Psychiatry 136:555–558, 1979

Weissman MM, Klerman GL, Prusoff BA, et al: Depressed outpatients: results one year after treatment with drugs and/or interpersonal psychotherapy. Arch Gen Psychiatry 38:52–55, 1981

Weissman MM, Rounsaville BJ, Chevron ES: Training psychotherapists to participate in psychotherapy outcome studies: identifying and dealing with the research requirement. Am J Psychiatry 139:1442–1446, 1982

Weissman MM, Jarrett R, Rush JA: Psychotherapy and its relevance to the pharmacotherapy of major depression: a decade later (1976–1985), in Psychopharmacology: A Generation of Progress. Edited by Meltzer HY. New York, Raven, 1987, pp 1059–1070

Chapter 5

Continuation Therapy for Unipolar Depression: The Case for Combined Treatment

Ellen Frank, Ph.D.
David J. Kupfer, M.D.
Janet Levenson, B.A.

Chapter 5

Continuation Therapy for Unipolar Depression: The Case for Combined Treatment

In the decade that followed the discovery of the tricyclic antidepressants, so much excitement was generated by clinicians' new-found ability to treat the acute episode of depression that little attention was paid to the observation that approximately one-half of depressed patients, even those treated successfully with tricyclics, went on to a relapsing or recurring course. The "rediscovery" of this feature of unipolar illness in the last several years has increased interest in the concepts of continuation and maintenance treatment. Although the difference between continuation and maintenance treatment may not always be clear in the literature or in the minds of treating clinicians, we argue that these are two distinct treatment phases, each with its own goal. Continuation treatment is carried out to prevent relapse into the acute episode, whereas maintenance treatment is intended to prevent new episodes in a patient known to have recurrent illness.

If, then, the goal of continuation treatment is the prevention of relapse into the acute episode, there seem to be several logical reasons why a combination of pharmacotherapy and psychotherapy in this phase of treatment might be considered. First, assuming that there were interpersonal or intrapsychic conflicts associated with the onset of the acute episode, the continuation phase—in which the patient's remitted state makes concentration, intellectual integration, and the testing of new behaviors possible—may be the ideal time to explore such conflicts in psychotherapy. Second, active involvement in

This work was funded in part by National Institute of Mental Health Grants MH-29618 and MH-30915 and by the John D. and Catherine T. MacArthur Foundation Network on the Psychobiology of Depression and Related Affective Disorders.

135

psychotherapy may serve to prevent the reemergence of psychosocial problems resolved in the acute treatment phase. Such problems, if they crop up again, could make the patient more vulnerable to relapse. If nothing else, psychotherapy may keep the patient more engaged in treatment than a simple medication check would and, thus, less likely to discontinue medication. Fourth, turning things around, the advantage to psychotherapy of continued pharmacotherapy is that it may keep symptoms suppressed, facilitating the patient's ability to participate in psychotherapy and, thus, to act on what he or she learns in the process.

BASIC RESEARCH AND CLINICAL QUESTIONS

For some of the reasons outlined above, continuation treatment has been very much underdiscussed and understudied. Nonetheless, it is possible to frame the basic questions surrounding continuation treatment, which would include, What is the period of continuation treatment? When does continuation treatment begin? When does it end? Is there a place for continuation treatment even with patients experiencing a first episode of depression? Specifically, with respect to combined treatment in continuation, it might well be asked whether once a patient is remitted, is there any advantage to continuing combined therapy if that was the acute treatment regimen or should only the pharmacotherapy be continued? If treatment was begun with drug alone, is there any advantage to adding psychotherapy? Finally, and perhaps most important, which patients are likely to benefit from combined continuation treatment?

Earlier Studies of Combined Continuation Treatment

The literature is almost devoid of empirical information regarding combined continuation treatment. Searching the literature for information on "combined continuation treatment," in fact, provides little more than clinical anecdotes. However, using current terminology, the first studies of "maintenance treatment" can be considered to be studies of continuation therapy. These include the Boston–New Haven Collaborative Study (Paykel et al. 1975; Weissman et al. 1974), in which there was a combined treatment cell. In this study, 150 depressed female outpatients, all of whom had been successfully treated (i.e., had achieved a 50% reduction on the Raskin Severity of Depression Scale [RSDS; Raskin et al. 1969]) for 1 month with amitriptyline, were entered into a three-by-two design with three drug conditions and two psychotherapy conditions. The two psychotherapy conditions consisted of a high-contact cell, in which patients were seen by psychiatric social workers one to two times a week, and a low-contact condition, which consisted of seeing a psychiatrist for a medication check and prescribing one time each month. The high-contact condition later evolved into interpersonal psychotherapy (Klerman et al. 1984). The three experimental drug conditions were begun after a 2-month transition phase. Thus, at that point, patients had been on amitriptyline for a total of 3 months. One-third of the group was continued on amitriptyline, the average dose being a little over 100 mg, one-third was continued on placebo, and one-third was assigned to a no-pill condition. The total length of the study after the first month of amitriptyline treatment was 8 months. Of the 150 patients who reached the point of randomization, 106 completed the study. Thirty-three (22%) of the patients relapsed, with significantly more relapses in the no-drug conditions, and 11 patients (7%) dropped out of the study. With respect to symptom return, Paykel et al. (1975) reported a significant advantage for active drug over placebo or no pill. They found no advantage for psychotherapy and no drug-psychotherapy interactions. With respect to social adjustment, Weissman et al. (1974) reported a significant advantage for psychotherapy. This advantage became apparent only at 6 and 8 months. They reported no advantage for drugs in terms of social adjustment and no interaction effects. Therefore, taking both symptoms and social adjustment into account, it could be concluded that the combined treatment was superior to the other five conditions. However, an inspection of the data presented in the Paykel et al. and Weissman et al. reports suggests that it is unlikely that the type of survival analysis typically conducted on the results of such studies today would indicate significantly longer survival time in the combined-treatment cell.

Data on Combined Continuation Treatment From the Maintenance Therapies in Recurrent Depression Protocol

Our own study of maintenance treatment in recurrent depression provides for a 20-week combined continuation treatment phase before the experimental maintenance phase (Figure 5-1). Although this continuation therapy phase is not experimental, it does provide empirical data on combined treatment carried out under conditions of relatively frequent and intense scrutiny.

Study design. After giving informed consent, patients between the ages of 21 and 65 who suffered from a current nonbipolar major depression, confirmed by interview with the Schedule for Affective Disorders and Schizophrenia (Spitzer and Endicott 1975), were entered into the maintenance therapies in recurrent depression protocol if the index episode was at least their third lifetime episode

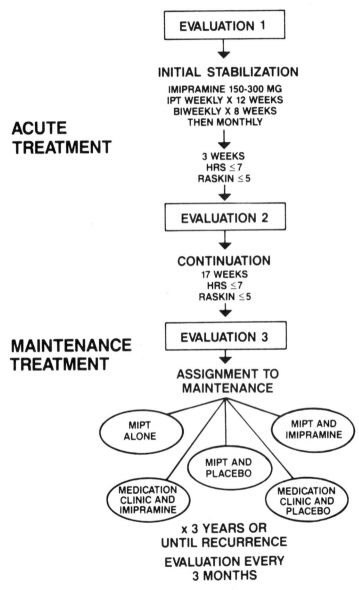

Figure 5-1. Maintenance therapies in recurrent depression study. IPT = interpersonal psychotherapy. HRS = Hamilton Rating Scale for Depression. MIPT = maintenance interpersonal psychotherapy.

of major unipolar depression. It was also necessary that the immediately preceding episode occurred no more than 2.5 years before the onset of the current one and that previous episodes required treatment or resulted in significant functional impairment. In addition, the patient was required to have minimum scores of 15 on the Hamilton Rating Scale for Depression (HRSD; Hamilton 1960) and 7 on the RSDS. Patients with primary diagnoses other than unipolar depression (e.g., alcoholism, phobic disorder, or panic disorder) were excluded, as were those who met DSM-III (American Psychiatric Association 1980) criteria for borderline or antisocial personality disorder. This last exclusion criterion obviously limits to some extent the range of personality traits and especially disorders to be found in our study population.

After a 2-week drug-free period, severity of depression was reevaluated, and patients who remained symptomatic were given a complete initial assessment including biological (all-night sleep EEG and neuroendocrine studies) and psychosocial (e.g., social adjustment and social support) measures. Because of the probable influence of acute illness on personality instruments (Hirschfeld et al. 1983), however, personality was not evaluated at this time.

All patients then received the same acute treatment regimen: imipramine (150–300 mg per day) and interpersonal psychotherapy (Klerman et al. 1984), offered weekly for 12 weeks, biweekly for 8 weeks, and monthly thereafter. At the point when patients had maintained a HRSD score of 7 or less and a RSDS score of 5 or less for 3 weeks, a second biological and psychosocial evaluation was completed. At this (continuation treatment) evaluation, personality was assessed for the first time with both self-report and interview measures (described below). Patients remained in continuation treatment for an additional 17 weeks, during which both HRSD and RSDS scores and imipramine dose were required to remain stable. A third (premaintenance) evaluation was then conducted, after which patients were randomly assigned to one of five maintenance treatments for 3 years or until they experienced a recurrence of illness. The five maintenance treatments consisted of 1) interpersonal psychotherapy (IPT) offered alone, 2) IPT offered with a placebo tablet, 3) IPT with active imipramine, 4) a medication clinic visit with a placebo tablet, or 5) a medication clinic visit with active imipramine.

Of the 230 patients who were entered into the acute treatment trial, 157 (68%) "stabilized," that is, achieved HRSD scores ≤7 and RSDS scores ≤5 for a period of 3 weeks. One hundred and twenty-eight of these 157 patients completed the remaining 17 weeks of continuation treatment. Twelve patients (7.6%) experienced a "relapse," defined as meeting criteria for major depressive disorder and having a HRSD score of at least 15 and a RSDS rating of at least 7, after at least 6 weeks of remission (HRSD ≤7; RSDS ≤5). Nine patients (5.7%) were discontinued from the study because of intolerable side effects or other complications of treatment, and 11 patients (7%) dropped out or were terminated for noncompliance. These figures compare quite favorably with continuation studies in which pharmacotherapy alone was used. For example, in the Mindham et al. (1973) study, 22% of the active drug–treated patients relapsed over the 6-month continuation treatment period.

Symptomatic exacerbations during continuation treatment: the "blip" phenomenon. Our original criterion for a clear-cut clinical remission and entry into the experimental maintenance phase was defined by the continuation treatment phase, which was to consist of 20 consecutive weeks of stable HRSD scores ≤7. In fact, this criterion proved too stringent for practical application. Whereas 81 (63%) of the 128 patients never experienced a HRSD score higher than 9 during the 20-week period, 26 patients (20%) experienced at least one symptomatic "blip" (HRSD >10) and 21 patients (16%) experienced two or more blips.

Table 5-1 shows the demographic and clinical characteristics of the three groups of patients. As can be seen, the population was predominantly female and middle-aged. Although only two previous episodes were required for entry into the protocol, most patients had had at least four earlier episodes, with the first episode occurring in their 20s. On average, the population had been symptomatic for approximately 6 months at the time of initial evaluation and was rated as moderately to severely ill for an outpatient population. The groups did not differ with respect to sex, age, number of previous episodes, duration of the index episode, age at onset of illness, or HRSD score at initial evaluation.

Not surprisingly, the patients who experienced symptomatic blips, both those experiencing only one and those experiencing more than one, differed significantly from the patients who experienced no blips in terms of their HRSD score at the last continuation evaluation. It also seems logical that these two groups of patients were being treated with a significantly higher dose of imipramine than were the patients who experienced no blips, especially in light of the acute treatment experience of these three groups of patients, which is described below. With respect to imipramine plasma levels, the 26 patients who experienced one blip had an imipramine plasma level that was significantly higher than that observed in the no-blip patients. Although

Table 5-1. Clinical characteristics of patients by "blip" grouping

Clinical characteristics	Number of "blips"		
	None ($n = 81$)	1 ($n = 26$)	≥ 2 ($n = 21$)
Sex			
Male	18 (22%)	7 (27%)	5 (24%)
Female	63 (78%)	19 (73%)	16 (76%)
Age (years)	41.63 ± 11.38	37.61 ± 10.53	38.05 ± 8.90
Number of previous episodes	6.85 ± 5.95	8.96 ± 12.02	4.14 ± 2.73
Age at onset (years)	27.86 ± 11.33	25.04 ± 9.17	26.67 ± 8.73
Duration of index episode (weeks)	23.24 ± 18.61	24.62 ± 20.06	24.91 ± 16.20
HRSD score at baseline	21.90 ± 4.89	20.62 ± 4.15	22.10 ± 4.89
HRSD score at last continuation	2.47 ± 2.27	5.92 ± 5.29	4.86 ± 4.89**
Imipramine dose (mg)	204.32 ± 65.65	237.50 ± 52.56	233.33 ± 74.30*
Imipramine plasma level (ng/ml)	268.39 ± 116.69	374.75 ± 120.63	296.41 ± 122.21*

Note. HRSD = Hamilton Rating Scale for Depression. Values are means ± SD.
*$P < .05$. **$P < .001$.

the two-or-more-blip group also appears to have an average dose higher than that of the no-blip group, it was not significantly higher. ***Does acute treatment course predict continuation treatment course?*** Having observed that the three patient groups differed significantly in certain aspects of the course of their continuation treatment, we next took a retrospective look to see whether the patients who had a smooth experience in continuation treatment differed from those who experienced blips in terms of their acute treatment experience.

Early in our study, we noted that some patients had a relatively rapid and sustained response to the combined acute treatment, whereas others responded more slowly (Frank et al. 1984; Frank et al. 1987). To quantify and describe this observation systematically, we developed an algorithm for categorizing patients according to acute treatment response (see Table 5-2). Although the majority of patients discussed here were categorized as either normal or slow responders, a smaller number of patients met neither the normal- nor the slow-responder criteria, but nonetheless were able to stabilize and were ultimately entered into the continuation phase. These patients were categorized as partial responders in the analysis of response during the first 16 weeks of combined acute treatment.

The no-blip group was significantly more likely to have had a normal response to acute treatment, whereas the one-blip group was about equally divided between normal and slow responders, (Table 5-3). The two-or-more-blip group included a majority of patients who were classified as either slow or partial responders.

Personality characteristics and the course of combined continuation treatment. Because we had previously found a relationship between personality features and response to acute treatment (Frank et al. 1987), we next examined personality features in the three blip group-

Table 5-2. Algorithm for determining acute treatment response type

HRSD score at			% change in HRSD score from baseline to 16 weeks	Type of responder
8 weeks	12 weeks	16 weeks		
≤7	<10	≤7	≥50	Normal
≤7	≥10	≤7	≥50	Slow
>7	≥0	8–10	≥60	Slow
Any patient who does not fit into above categories				Partial or nonresponder

HRSD = Hamilton Rating Scale for Depression.

ings, with the expectation that patients with a more variable course of continuation treatment might be expected to show more personality disturbance. To assess personality, patients were evaluated with the Personality Assessment Form (PAF) developed for the Treatment of Depression Collaborative Research Project (Shea et al. 1987). The PAF provides continuous scores from 0 to 6 on all 11 of the DSM-III personality disorder categories as well as a rating for dysthymia. It was administered at both the beginning and end of the continuation treatment phase by the subjects' primary therapist. Data from the second PAF evaluation were used in the present analysis. Only dependency (χ^2 = 5.98, df 2; P = .05) and dysthymia (χ^2 = 10.48 df 2; P = .005) were found to differ significantly across the three blip groupings. The two-or-more-blip group was significantly more likely to be rated in the 4–6 range (probable or definite disorder) on both dependency and dysthymia. Needless to say, the fact that clinicians tended to view those patients with more symptomatic exacerbations during continuation treatment as more like those individuals who meet criteria for dysthymia is no surprise.

Biological characteristics and the course of combined continuation treatment. We were also curious about the extent to which these three groups of patients might differ with respect to baseline biological parameters. We therefore examined a selected group of EEG sleep features in these patients. There were significant differences observed across the three groups, but only with respect to rapid-eye-movement (REM) sleep (Table 5-4). In the manually scored sleep, there was a trend (P = .065) for baseline REM activity to be lower in the one- and two-blip groups. This finding reached statistical significance (P < .05) in the analysis of average REM counts derived from automated

Table 5-3. Acute treatment response of three "blip" groupings

	Number of "blips"		
	None (n = 78)[a]	1 (n = 25)[a]	≥2 (n = 21)
Normal responder	46 (57%)	10 (38%)	3 (14%)
Slow responder	23 (28%)	10 (38%)	15 (71%)
Partial or nonresponder	9 (11%)	5 (19%)	3 (14%)

Note. χ^2 = 15.85, df 4; P = .003.
[a]Three patients in the no-blip group and one patient in the one-blip group could not be classified in terms of their acute treatment response.

Table 5-4. Baseline sleep EEG by "blip" grouping

	Number of "blips"		
	None	1	≥2
Manual scoring			
Sleep latency (minutes)	27.10 ± 21.64	24.10 ± 17.12	21.88 ± 15.59
Sleep maintenance (%)	91.10 ± 7.87	93.67 ± 6.95	93.41 ± 6.94
REM latency (minutes)	72.31 ± 36.67	83.69 ± 37.47	78.71 ± 25.55
REM activity (units)**	110.94 ± 44.22	105.54 ± 57.49	86.69 ± 57.82
Percentage of stage 1	6.05 ± 4.76	5.57 ± 3.12	7.42 ± 5.38
Automated scoring			
Total delta (counts)	2585.01 ± 1650.7	2604.89 ± 1070.83	2932.45 ± 2209.75
Total REM (counts)	9.51 ± 5.87	9.26 ± 3.78	10.45 ± 7.42
Average delta (counts)	729.44 ± 406.36	717.83 ± 510.93	546.03 ± 442.72
Average REM (counts)*	7.88 ± 4.14	6.98 ± 3.78	5.35 ± 2.98

Note. REM = rapid eye movement. Values are means ± SD.
*$P < .05$. **$P = .065$.

scoring, which indicated significantly less REM in the two-or-more-blip group. This appears to suggest that the REM features of the no-blip group are more typical of endogenous major depressive disorder, whereas the patients who went on to experience a variable course in combined continuation treatment had REM features that were less prototypic of the sleep of individuals with major depression. *Social adjustment and the course of combined continuation treatment.* We were also curious as to whether social adjustment, as measured either at the beginning or the end of continuation treatment, might differ among these three groups of patients. We examined data from the Social Adjustment Scale—II interview (Schooler et al. 1980). Significant differences were observed across groups when a simple repeated measures analysis of variance was conducted on Social Adjustment Scale scores. However, because in all of our analyses we found that HRSD scores and Social Adjustment Scale scores were highly correlated and because our blip groupings were entirely dependent on HRSD scores, we concluded that the only meaningful analysis of social adjustment data was one in which we controlled for HRSD scores. These analyses are displayed in Tables 5-5 and 5-6. When we controlled for HRSD scores, all group effects disappeared; however, both work adjustment and social-leisure adjustment showed significant improvement over time and parental role adjustment showed a significant interaction effect, with the no-blip group improving on parental role adjustment, whereas the one-blip and two-or-more-blip groups deteriorated over the period of continuation treatment. Only modest credence should be given to this finding because a reduced number of subjects were rated on the parental role and a large number of analyses were run.

Does the course of continuation treatment predict recurrence of illness? Finally, and perhaps most important, we examined the experience of these three groups of patients in the maintenance phase of our study. Because we know that, at least for the first 18 months of the maintenance phase, the different maintenance treatments have significantly different survival rates associated with them (Frank et al. 1989), we examined the three blip groupings' experience in maintenance treatment controlling for their maintenance treatment assignment; we found absolutely no differences with respect to survival time in maintenance. In other words, those patients who experienced no symptomatic exacerbations during continuation treatment had neither longer nor shorter survival time than those who experienced such exacerbations during the continuation treatment phase. The course of combined continuation treatment thus does not appear to have predictive value with respect to new episodes of major depression.

SUMMARY

Clearly, few definitive conclusions can be drawn about combined continuation treatment; however, the data do provide some hints. It appears that combined continuation treatment keeps relapse at a minimum, particularly when drug dose is adequate. The 7.6% relapse rate observed in our combined continuation phase compares quite favorably with the 12–48% rate observed in active drug studies (Ayd 1979). It also appears that combined continuation has an advantage in terms of keeping patients engaged in treatment. Only 7% of the patients engaged in this continuation phase dropped out or needed to be terminated for noncompliance.

Table 5-5. Social Adjustment Scale scores for three "blip" groupings at beginning and end of continuation treatment

	Number of "blips"		
Role area	None	1	≥2
Work			
Beginning	2.13 ± .70	2.35 ± .56	2.50 ± .51
End	1.67 ± .57	2.19 ± .75	2.05 ± .51
Social/leisure			
Beginning	2.30 ± .63	2.32 ± .80	2.79 ± .85
End	1.89 ± .62	2.32 ± .80	2.37 ± .76
Extended family			
Beginning	2.38 ± .76	2.24 ± .78	2.31 ± .60
End	2.17 ± .71	2.20 ± .71	2.38 ± .50
Principal household member			
Beginning	2.11 ± .70	2.13 ± .64	2.50 ± 1.00
End	1.82 ± .73	2.00 ± .65	2.17 ± .83
Parental			
Beginning	2.26 ± .86	2.20 ± .63	2.20 ± .63
End	1.87 ± .67	2.40 ± .69	2.30 ± .48
Overall			
Beginning	2.32 ± .62	2.60 ± .65	2.70 ± .66
End	2.00 ± .65	2.40 ± .87	2.55 ± .69

Note. Values are means ± SD.

Table 5-6. Repeated measures analysis of variance (ANOVA) and analysis of covariance (ANCOVA) on Social Adjustment Scale scores obtained at beginning and end of continuation treatment

Global score	Repeated-measures ANOVA			Repeated-measures ANOVA covaried for HRSD		
	Group	Time	Interaction	Global	Time	Interaction
Work	$F = 8.71$ $P = .0003$	28.37 .0001	1.43 2.443	$F = 1.91$ $P = .1528$	11.14 .0011	0.98 .3771
Social	$F = 6.19$ $P = .0028$	17.87 .0001	2.35 .0996	$F = 2.65$ $P = .0751$	4.28 .0407	2.20 .1153
Extended family	$F = 0.21$ $P = .8117$	3.23 .0750	1.00 .3700	$F = 1.03$ $P = .3607$	0.50 .8167	1.31 .2752
Household member	$F = 2.01$ $P = .1413$	7.08 .0094	0.20 .8172	$F = 0.32$ $P = .7244$	0.86 .3574	0.36 .7008
Parental	$F = 0.77$ $P = .4670$	2.55 .1166	2.86 .0671	$F = 0.05$ $P = .9507$	0.12 .7345	3.91 .0504
Overall	$F = 8.82$ $P = .0003$	11.48 .0010	0.38 .6819	$F = 2.16$ $P = .1203$	1.52 .2197	0.85 .4315

Note. HRSD = Hamilton Rating Scale for Depression.

It is highly probable that each treatment reinforces the other. Continued symptom suppression through continued medication probably facilitates participation in psychotherapy. Continued participation in psychotherapy probably reduces vulnerability to relapse through mechanisms we do not yet fully understand.

The data described in this chapter also provide several leads as to future studies that might be helpful. It would certainly be important to compare a group of patients who are continued on their acute treatment dose of medication with patients who are continued on a somewhat-reduced dose, both with and without continued psychotherapy. It would also be important to test various frequencies of psychotherapeutic contact in combination with pharmacotherapy. At this point, we do not know what frequency of psychotherapeutic contact provides the best cost-benefit ratio for continuation treatment. Finally, and this applies to all types of continuation studies including drug therapy, psychotherapy, and combined treatment studies, the field is clearly in need of investigations that would lead to data on the ideal length of continuation treatment when the prevention of relapse is the goal.

REFERENCES

American Psychiatric Association: Diagnostic and Statistical Manual of Mental Disorders, 3rd Edition. Washington, DC, American Psychiatric Association, 1980

Ayd FJ: Continuation and maintenance doxepin (Sinequan) therapy: ten years' experience. International Drug Therapy Newsletter 14:3–4, 1979

Frank E, Jarrett DB, Kupfer DJ, et al: Biological and clinical predictors of response in recurrent depression (a preliminary report). Psychiatry Res 13:315–324, 1984

Frank E, Kupfer DJ, Jacob M, et al: Personable features and response to acute treatment in recurrent depression. Journal of Personality Disorders 1:14–26, 1987

Frank E, Kupfer DJ, Perel JM: Early recurrence in unipolar depression. Arch Gen Psychiatry 46:397–400, 1989

Hamilton M: A rating scale for depression. J Neurol Neurosurg Psychiatry 23:56–62, 1960

Hirschfeld RM, Klerman GL, Clayton PJ, et al: Assessing personality: effects of the depressive state on trait measurement. Psychiatry 140:695–699, 1983

Klerman GL, Weissman MM, Rounsaville BJ, et al: Interpersonal Psychotherapy of Depression. New York, Basic Books, 1984

Mindham RHS, Howland C, Shepherd M: An evaluation of continuation therapy with tricyclic antidepressants in depressive illness. Psychol Med 3:5–17, 1973

Paykel ES, DiMascio A, Haskell D, et al: Effects of maintenance amitriptyline and psychotherapy on symptoms of depression. Psychol Med 5:67–77, 1975

Raskin A, Schulterbrandt J, Reatig N, et al: Replication of factors of psychopathology in interview, ward behavior, and self-report ratings of hospitalized depressives. J Nerv Ment Dis 148:87–98, 1969

Schooler NR, Levine G, Severe JB, et al: Prevention of relapse and schizophrenia: an evaluation of fluphenazine decanoate. Arch Gen Psychiatry 37:16–25, 1980

Shea MT, Glass DR, Pilkonis PA, et al: Frequency and implications of personality disorders in a sample of depressed outpatients. Journal of Personality Disorders 1:27–42, 1987

Spitzer RL, Endicott J: Schedule for Affective Disorders and Schizophrenia. New York, New York State Psychiatric Institute, 1975

Weissman M, Klerman GL, Paykel ES, et al: Treatment effects on the social adjustment of depressed patients. Arch Gen Psychiatry 30:771–778, 1974

Chapter 6

Combined Psychotherapeutic and Psychopharmacologic Treatment of Depressed Patients: Clinical Observations

Carl Salzman, M.D.
Jules Bemporad, M.D.

Chapter 6

Combined Psychotherapeutic and Psychopharmacologic Treatment of Depressed Patients: Clinical Observations

Most contemporary psychiatrists would agree that depression may result from dysregulated central nervous system function, from psychological or interpersonal stresses, or from both. Uncertainty over determining the etiology of depression is further compounded by distinctions between depressions of different severity, bipolar versus unipolar depressions, and depressions that may arise in relation to other illness or symptoms, as compared with autonomous, primary depressions. Unfortunately, depressions of different etiologies do not have different clinical manifestations, and typically depressed patients usually have evidence of both neurobiologic and psychologic dysfunction.

Despite the lack of discriminating features, psychiatrists in clinical practice commonly endeavor to differentiate depressions that have a neurobiologic basis from those that are more psychologic in origin, believing that medication is more appropriate for the former and psychotherapy for the latter. There is little evidence to support such an etiological subdivision, and little evidence to suggest that psychotherapy is useful for one form of depression whereas psychopharmacology is more suitable for the other. In fact, treatment response to antidepressant drugs is predicted almost exclusively by pretreatment symptom pattern (assuming adequate dose and duration of drug treatment) and not by etiology, nor presence or absence of precipitating stress. However, successful reduction of depressive symptoms does not, by itself, always constitute successful treatment of depression—psychological factors may still require psychological treatment.

It is our thesis in this chapter that for patients who are seriously depressed (i.e., have major depressive disorder), neither psychopharmacologic treatment alone nor psychotherapeutic treatment alone is appropriate or sufficient. Rather, we argue that both treatments are necessary and augment the other's therapeutic effect. Our comments are based on clinical experience as opposed to a review of the literature.

DIAGNOSTIC CRITERIA FOR DEPRESSION

Psychiatric treatment should follow diagnostic precision. In past years, psychodynamically oriented diagnoses emphasized developmental and premorbid history, as well as the presence or absence of familial and intrapsychic conflict. Acute symptoms were understood as only a recent manifestation of longer-standing psychopathology, usually extending back to childhood (i.e., clinical depression as the tip of a psychological iceberg found from depressive psychosocial development). Contemporary diagnostic criteria, primarily utilizing DSM-III-R (American Psychiatric Association 1987) and related classification schemes, have reversed this trend. Now, current symptom clusters are relied on entirely for the diagnosis, and long-standing or preexisting developmental or personality disorders are only utilized as adjunctive diagnostic classifications rather than as an essential ingredient of the primary diagnosis. This emphasis on a cross-sectional diagnostic scheme does not address a common clinical situation; depressed patients, in addition to their classic symptoms of depression, often suffer as well from such problems as irrational or excessive guilt, pathological interpersonal relationships, impaired ability to love, an inability to function to one's full level of capabilities, an overreaction to the emotional buffeting of daily life, an impaired ability to impart self-esteem to others, especially one's children, and, most significantly, an impaired sense of one's own self-worth and of belonging in the world. Clinical experience suggests that these symptoms often antedate the onset of the clinical depression and may persist even after clinical depression has resolved and possibly predispose the person to future relapses.

Antidepressant drugs, given in proper doses for adequate periods of time, have been repeatedly demonstrated to treat the classic symptoms of major depressive disorder. However, it has been our experience that even when these symptoms of acute depression have abated, some patients are still left with a psychological, subjective experience of unhappiness and low self-esteem. It is important to emphasize that even patients who return to a life that is highly functional and are objectively completely free from depressive symptoms may nevertheless still suffer from extreme inner unhappiness. Such self-dissatisfaction, often long-standing, may, in fact, be a central feature of some people's identity. It is not clear whether these people are more predisposed to depression, or more vulnerable to relapse after a remitted depression. We believe, however, that such people are less resilient to normal life stress and, when depressed, require more than symptom reduction for adequate treatment.

Antidepressant drugs are less consistently useful for these inner experiences of unhappiness. It is our clinical observation that the antidepressant pharmacologic effects and the psychotherapeutic psychologic effects are directed toward different aspects of clinical symptoms. Antidepressant drugs clearly are more effective for symptom reduction and for prophylaxis of carefully defined depressive episodes (as reflected in depressive rating scale score reductions). Psychotherapy, in contrast, focuses not on the clinical symptom picture of major depression, but on the inner subjective dissatisfaction that is usually not responsive to antidepressants. We further hypothesize that these inner psychologic features may predispose the patient to recurrence of clinical depressive episodes, especially in those who also may have a neurobiologic and genetic vulnerability to depression. Psychotherapy, in these cases, is not a specific treatment for depression, but a means of improving the patient's means of coping with his or her inner life and with external experiences. By strengthening the individual's ability to judge himself or herself and others in a realistic adult manner, the vulnerability to depression may be lessened as more adaptive and flexible responses to anticipated life stressors are mastered.

NATURE OF THE DEPRESSED PATIENT

Predisposition to Depression

If one talks carefully with people who are clinically depressed, one is impressed that the depression rarely strikes "out of the blue," i.e., without observable antecedents. Unlike pneumonia, which may suddenly afflict someone with no prior pulmonary disease, it is our observation that depression is most frequently seen in patients who have a psychological as well as a biological predisposition to depression before the onset of a clinical episode. The biological vulnerability may be inferred from a family history that is positive for major affective disorder. The psychological predisposition may be less obvious: a history of past loss, childhood or parental difficulties, unrequited loves, unfulfilled expectations, or inaccurate self-appraisals.

The relationship between depression and intercurrent difficulties in psychological functioning is well known. Sometimes called "double depression" (Keller and Shapiro 1982) or characterological depression (Akiskal 1983), some patients experience a pessimistic, gloomy, dysphoric outlook on life, even when not clinically depressed as defined by either research or clinical (DSM) criteria. At least 12–15% of individuals who have experienced a clinical episode of depression will fail to recover completely and will continue to experience significant depressive symptomatology for years or until a new decompensation occurs (Scott 1988). Although the reason for this chronicity may depend on many factors, it has been observed repeatedly that individuals with certain premorbid personality traits are more prone to chronic depressive symptoms and to failure in response to traditional treatment. For example, people with rigorous criteria for their own moral conduct, as well as for the conduct of others, and who may have exacting standards regarding behavior, performance, and hygiene, may be represented with unusual frequency among those who develop clinical depressions. Equally common among chronically or episodically depressed individuals are those with excessive needs for dependence on others and who have great difficulty in maintaining their psychic equilibrium without a sustaining relationship. For example, in one study of depressed women, there were fewer confiding close relationships, less employment outside the home, a greater presence of three or more young children in the household, and a history of maternal loss in childhood than in nondepressed women (Brown and Harris 1978). These factors were interpreted as reducing the individual's capacity to deal adequately with a threat to one's sense of security or self-esteem. Treatment of symptoms alone would not alter this inability to cope with the necessary losses and frustration of human experience.

Rather than depending entirely on the concepts of "double depression," or "characterological depression," we prefer to conceptualize the personality of some depressed individuals with a more commonplace term like "unhappy" or "dissatisfied." As we have commented, this term would apply to people who are not clinically depressed, who are often functional, and who by most clinical criteria could not be defined as sick or impaired. Nevertheless, by their own subjective standards, they are dissatisfied, pessimistic, inhibited, unhappy, and gloomy and feel unfulfilled by their daily lives. Often these dissatisfactions are long-standing and extend into the person's own interpersonal function, sexual function, or sense of self-worth and capacity to love and be loved, etc. Despite external trappings of success such as seemingly successful jobs and family life, such patients may continue to experience life as dysphoric, threatening, and uncertain.

When these characteristics intensify, they may meet the criteria for true clinical depression.

Symptoms

It is our opinion that there are two components to depressive illness and thus two components to treatment. First, the symptom pattern of depression, as currently defined by research and clinical criteria, can be understood as a manifestation of altered central nervous system function in a genetically predisposed individual. Depressive episodes result from periodic malfunction in the brain's regulation of affect. However, we also conceptualize some of these patients as being vulnerable to life's stresses because of impaired psychological (character) formation, early childhood experiences, the nature of primary attachments to parents, and the nature of repeated experiences of success or failure. In such patients, depression can be understood as the result of life stresses interacting with a psychological vulnerability, perhaps in the presence of a genetically determined biological predisposition. It is our position that for such patients, neither antidepressant treatment alone nor psychotherapy alone is sufficient, and psychotherapy must be employed, together with antidepressant drugs.

Patients who are depressed usually present for treatment in one of two basic ways. One group may identify the source of their distress as outside themselves and identify events in their lives as a precipitant for the depression, such as loss of a loved one, job, skill, goal, etc; or they may focus entirely on physical factors such as illness or may magnify minor physical symptoms to explain their disturbed affect. For purposes of discussion, we shall label these patients *medically (externally) oriented depressed patients*. Because the source of affective distress is located outside themselves, then the usual request to the physician is for a treatment outside themselves, to reduce the symptoms. For such patients, antidepressant medications alone may be sufficiently therapeutic. Any attempt to place the depressive symptoms in a personal context of past history, current stress, or psychological conflict may be considered interesting but irrelevant. Psychotherapy makes no sense for these patients, because there is nothing to discuss except the severity of the symptoms and their response to the medication. For these medically oriented patients, psychotherapy, therefore, is limited to an interpersonal communication between doctor and patient, primarily serving to encourage and reinforce the appropriate taking of medication. Indeed, for some of these patients, the main psychotherapeutic task is to encourage the patient to remain on the medication long enough after symptom relief is attained so that rapid relapse is unlikely.

The other group of depressed patients identifies their depressive experience quite differently. Although the precipitant for the depressive episode may be a stress located in the environment outside the patient, it is clear that there exists within themselves either a vulnerability or predisposition to depression. Such people, for example, may describe fragile self-esteem, continual irrational feelings of guilt or concern over others' opinions, real or imagined failures to achieve personal goals, and frequent problems with intimate relationships. For such people, the emergence of a clinical depression is just a temporal exaggeration period of their usual feelings, or an intensification of affective experience that is consonant with their own self-understanding. We call these patients *psychologically (inwardly) oriented.*

It has been our impression that the presence of symptoms of depression in these psychologically oriented depressed patients may serve to propel the patient toward psychotherapeutic treatment, seeking more than just symptomatic relief. Not infrequently, these psychologically oriented patients question the efficacy of antidepressant treatment for long-standing psychologic or interpersonal problems; some may reject the use of antidepressants as too superficial. Others sometimes express the concern that use of medications indicates further evidence of their own inability to correct their psychological problems.

PSYCHOLOGIC MEANING OF ANTIDEPRESSANT MEDICATION

For many people, taking medication, especially one that alters subjective affective experience, may have psychological significances that transcend any specific pharmacological drug effect. These may be categorized as 1) the significance of the medical model and doctor-patient relationship, 2) the significance of healing factors outside the patient, and 3) the symbolic meaning of medication.

Doctor-Patient Relationship

As already discussed, the establishment of an empathic alliance between depressed patient and prescribing physician is one of the foundations of successful combined psychopharmacologic-psychotherapeutic treatment. It is not necessary, however, for the drug prescriber to be the therapist. If the patient understands that a nonprescribing therapist is sensitive to the signs indicating a need for medication, then a separation between therapist and prescriber is not antitherapeutic. Obvious problems arise when there is a disagreement between the therapist and prescriber regarding the need for medication. This disagreement may symbolically or actually represent splits in the patient between important past emotional figures into "good" and "bad," e.g., "caring" and "not caring." Some patients will see the prescribing physician as the powerful yet dangerous adult figure to be feared but obeyed, whereas the therapist becomes the empathic, understanding, but powerless caregiver. Other patients may interpret disagreements between therapist and prescriber in the opposite manner: the therapist does not care enough to take the patient's symptoms seriously, whereas the prescriber is the magical figure who truly understands the depth and extent of the patient's suffering. Of course, if there is a real disagreement between therapist and prescriber, then power struggles and countertherapeutic behavior may also occur, independent of the patient's true needs. It is critical, therefore, for therapist and prescriber to communicate and discuss any differences in therapeutic perspectives or goals for the patient. For patients who may be especially vulnerable to distinctions between caring and not-caring transference figures, a single therapist-prescriber may be preferable.

Healing Factors Outside the Patient

For some patients, especially those who need to maintain tight control over their behavior and affect, the taking of medication may be interpreted as surrendering control. Not only do the pharmacological effects of the drug remove affective experience from personal control, but such control is then placed in the hands of a prescriber, who, therefore, becomes quite powerful and potentially dangerous. For such patients, the cultivation of a trusting, empathic alliance is necessary before they may entirely accept the role of medication. During the early phases of treatment of a depression, when symptoms are severe, this trust is less critical than in the subsequent phases when symptom resolution is less urgent. As the depression resolves, the patient may begin to question the wisdom of the medication prescription and, by inference, the trust in the prescribing physician. It is not unusual to hear patients express doubt about the original necessity for antidepressant medication, and even question the accuracy of the diagnosis or the assessment of the severity of the depression. Without a firm trusting alliance, such patients may discontinue medication or not take the drugs as prescribed and risk relapse.

Symbolic Meaning of Medication

During a phase of psychologic regression, when a depressed patient's functioning shifts back toward a state of greater dependence, the pill that will bring symptomatic relief may be experienced as an incorporation of the "good mother," or trusted adult figure. Because most antidepressant medications are taken orally, the pills may also represent a symbolic feeding and therefore a form of nurturance, and result in tension reduction. Some patients may even experience antidepressant drug effect before the pharmacologic effect of any drug is possible, and such symptom relief may be explained by the symbolic power of the medication. As most physicians know, therefore, the strength of a drug's healing powers depends partly on the nature of the therapeutic relationship between doctor and patient. For the depressed patient who trusts the prescribing physician in the context of a warm, empathic alliance, the antidepressant drug may become a concrete piece of the therapist that is taken in, as nourishment is taken in from a parent by the young (or regressed) individual who cannot care for himself or herself. The antidepressant drug also represents a concrete demonstration by the physician that the patient's symptoms are taken seriously, and that further worsening is not necessary to attract the caregiver's attention.

DEFINITION OF PSYCHOTHERAPY

We define psychotherapy as an interpersonal relationship, involving communication between patient and therapist that has certain characteristics and is based on certain conceptual premises. It is necessary to define these clinical and conceptual factors in order to discuss the therapeutic role of psychotherapy in depression.

Psychotherapy exerts its effect by a process of self-discovery and a careful exploration of those events that have left their mark on the adult personality. This long-term process is one in which the patient is a consenting participant, having made the decision to work with a therapist for an extended period. Such an important choice should be arrived at after symptomatic relief has been achieved and not forced on an individual who in the search for a surcease from pain will agree to any form of treatment. It is also imperative in initiating any form of treatment to separate those aspects of personality malfunction that are the result rather than the cause of a depressive episode.

The type of psychotherapy that will be discussed in this chapter can be termed *intensive psychodynamic* or *psychoanalytically oriented psychotherapy*. This form of therapy relies heavily on discovering and altering those personality patterns that are believed to increase the individual's vulnerability to clinical illness. It is assumed that these characteristic modes of assessing oneself and others, of obtaining a sense of worth or self-esteem, or of inhibiting or gratifying one's desires were established in the individual's experience with significant others in childhood. These patterns of activity, feeling, and thinking become automatic in adult life although some originally served the purpose of avoiding the pain of abandonment or criticism or for obtaining the pleasure of security or praise from parents and other important figures. Although possibly adaptive in childhood, these outmoded personality patterns no longer are appropriate to adult life but persist nevertheless, often without the awareness of the individual. In intensive psychotherapy, these inappropriate patterns are identified, sometimes with considerable discomfort, in the context of current relationships or beliefs, with the goal of eventually substituting more reality-based forms of inner, as well as interpersonal, functioning. Much of therapy, therefore, consists of identifying, examining, and correcting the results of one's upbringing that interfere with the responsibilities and rewards of adult life.

COMBINED PSYCHOPHARMACOLOGY AND PSYCHOTHERAPY

Early Phase

In the early phase of treatment, when the patient's depressive symptoms are serious enough to compromise normal function, all treatment efforts are directed exclusively toward symptom reduction. In this phase, patients often do not have enough mental (or even physical) energy to enter into a true psychotherapeutic relationship. They tend to focus on dystonic symptoms, express feelings of hopelessness and pointlessness, and may even have trouble concentrating on a spoken dialogue between themselves and their therapist. Accompanying these severe symptoms of psychomotor depletion is the common wish to be taken care of ("regress"); patients in this phase of depression often complain that they are unable to participate actively in any kind of therapeutic process and wish to be left alone. Discussion of prior negative experiences or inner unhappiness only add to the experience of overwhelming depression.

For the medically oriented patient, expressions of physical discomfort or unrealistic concern with physical health or minor physical ailments dominate all thoughts and conversation. Psychotherapy at this early phase is not really possible. As noted by Semrad, this is the phase of symptom resolution, rather than restructuring. ("If a house is on fire as a result of faulty electrical wiring, the first task is to put out the fire, not rewire the house.")

The primary treatment is antidepressant therapy. There are two categories of antidepressant effects that may prove useful in this early phase of the treatment of depressions. First is the pharmacological antidepressant effect, which usually begins after several days or weeks of treatment. Given a correct diagnosis of depression, and the use of appropriate doses of an antidepressant for a sufficient period, approximately 80% of nonpsychotic patients with major depressive disorder will experience clinically significant relief. Although there may be substantial side effects, most recovering patients are quite grateful for the relief of their primary depressive symptoms.

A second consequence of antidepressant treatment is more subtle and is not specifically related to symptom reduction. Antidepressants may energize the psychologically depleted and demoralized patient. This energy enhances the treatment by augmenting motivation while waiting for the pharmacologic antidepressant effect. This energizing function, noted many years ago by Ostow (1962), also provides the fuel required for psychotherapeutic work in later stages of combined treatment.

Psychotherapy plays three critical roles in this early treatment phase. First, psychotherapy may reinforce the administration of appropriate antidepressant therapy. Because some depressed patients are so nihilistic ("Don't bother with me, doctor, I'm not worth treating"), they may refuse to take medications or not take them as prescribed. Empathic psychotherapeutic communication between prescribing physician and suffering patient can make a critical difference in whether adequate antidepressant therapy is achieved.

The second major role for psychotherapy in this early treatment phase is preparatory. By establishing an empathic therapeutic alliance during the time of most intense suffering, the therapist becomes identified as an accepting and caring individual who may be trusted during times of pain and regression. It is this early establishment of a therapeutic alliance that will later serve as the substrate for ongoing psychotherapy as the depressive symptoms resolve.

The third role of psychotherapy is to teach the patient to look inward and to become conscious of particular vulnerabilities that may have contributed to the depressive episode. These vulnerabilities often emerge as atavistic patterns of self-evaluation or participation in relationships of which the individual may have only dimly perceived, if at all. Bringing these patterns to light and anchoring them in present psychosocial interchanges as well as in childhood modes of behavior begins to allow the individual to evaluate his or her life and to appraise more realistically the sources of gratification, need to please the dictates of others, past inhibitions, and, not infrequently, secret hatred and envy toward others. In this manner, the patient is taught to observe his or her own thoughts and actions and to see their connection to his or her ongoing discomfort. As the patient becomes more self-aware, he or she can start to consider the currently dysfunctional nature of reactions based on belief systems internalized during the formative childhood years. As the individual becomes more "psychologically minded" with the therapist's guidance, psychotherapy has truly been initiated. Looking inward, the patient attempts to link the precipitating stressor(s) to areas of psychological vulnerability and everyday mode of personality functioning. In this manner, the patient, with the help of the therapist, realizes this prior need to repress affects, to continue in unsuccessful forms of relationships, and to assess worth in an unrealistic manner.

Middle Phase

As antidepressant treatment begins to ameliorate depressive symptoms, the psychotherapeutic relationship plays another critical therapeutic role. It is in this phase of early recovery, when depressive symptoms are still present but energy is being restored, that patients are at the greatest risk for self-destructive behavior. As most clinicians know, it is dangerous for therapists to express too much optimism about the progress in symptomatic relief, because such comments may be misinterpreted by the still partially depressed patient as a wish on the psychiatrist's part to reject or dismiss the patient. This perceived rejection may be further misinterpreted as evidence supporting the patient's own harsh and critical self-judgment ("I really am a bad person . . . and deserve to die"). The task of the psychotherapist, at this middle phase, is to continue to emphasize the empathic alliance, sometimes by simply continuing to see the patient as frequently as during the earlier acute phases of the illness. Within this alliance, the psychiatrist emphasizes the need for continued medication. For medically oriented patients, careful and realistic discussions of drug side effects may serve to reinforce the medical nature of the doctor-patient relationship.

The Onset of Psychotherapy

As the depressive symptoms continue to resolve and the patient resumes normal functioning, psychotherapeutic examination of aspects of the patient's inner and past life may begin to be explored. At this phase, the patient has enough mental and physical energy to engage in an ongoing dialogue with the therapist and has enough motivation to continue therapeutic work from session to session. This is the beginning of the "rewiring of the house." Regression has ended, and preoccupation with symptoms has lessened sufficiently to allow the patient to consider other aspects of his or her experience. In psychopharmacologic terms, the antidepressant drug therapy has been successful, ratings of depressive symptoms have plummeted, and the depression is resolving.

It is in this phase of symptom resolution that true psychotherapy begins. As one patient commented: "The drugs cleared away the underbrush [depressive symptoms] making it possible to more clearly see the issues for therapy." Preoccupation with depressive symptoms has subsided, and the patient and therapist now continue with greater emphasis the task of identifying characterologic factors that may have been associated with the development of a depression. These include childhood and past experiences, character formation, interpersonal functioning, tolerance of affect, and accurate self-appraisal. Psychotherapeutic work in this early resolution phase must be delicate; the patient is not yet entirely healed. Even patients who wish to deny or avoid thinking of their depressive pain are vulnerable to return of symptoms. Psychotherapeutic exploration of prior unhappiness, therefore, must be conducted gently, and in the context of the ongoing supportive empathic alliance. It is helpful to continue to emphasize the therapeutic role of antidepressants in order to reinforce the "medical model" and the recognition that the therapist is concerned about present and recent unhappiness as well as past experience. Furthermore, it is usually critical for patients to continue their antidepressant drug treatment during this phase; premature tapering of the dose or discontinuation may lead to a relapse. Thus, the therapist now has the dual role of encouraging the patient to continue the treatment that brought about symptom relief, at the same time gently asking the patient to consider those aspects of his or her character that may have either predisposed the patient toward developing a depression or made the patient vulnerable to life stresses so that the biological inherited predisposition to depression was activated. As another patient commented, the fog has lifted, revealing the landscape underneath.

A third function of psychotherapy during this early resolution phase is to help guide the patient back into normal adult autonomy and functioning. For patients who have psychologically regressed during their depressive episode, especially those who required hospitalization or who were unable to work, attend school, or participate in usual daily activities, the therapist is challenged with the delicate task of encouraging a return to active life while acknowledging the presence of a biological-psychological defect that predisposed the patient to depression during previous normal functioning. Simple reassurance ("positive thinking") is not consistently helpful and is sometimes countertherapeutic because it may deny a reality known to both patient and therapist: a serious depression has just passed, and another may follow, because all the elements that caused the depression are still present. Reassurance may undermine the careful establishment of an empathic therapeutic alliance based on the mutual understanding that a severe decompensation was present, but that the patient was, nevertheless, still acceptable to the therapist. Reassurance may also signal to the patient a waning interest on the part of the therapist ("Why would he/she continue to be interested in me if I am feeling better?"). Therapist pessimism, or dire predictions of recurrent future depressions, on the other hand, also do not serve to enhance the therapeutic alliance and may activate the nihilistic fantasy (often expressed during the symptomatic peak of the depression) that all treatment efforts are useless. The patient must not come to perceive the therapist as sympathetic, which implies a recognition of patient defectiveness. Rather, the therapist must be experienced as empathic, as understanding and accepting of the patient's underlying predispositions to depression.

Maintaining a balance between encouraging cautious reentry into life as the depression resolves, supporting continuing drug treatment, and beginning to explore a patient's characterologic style and inner affective experience define the delicate therapeutic work that commences as the patient begins to feel less depressed.

Working Through

As the working-through phase of therapy commences, maladaptive beliefs have been identified. The task now is to demonstrate how they affect significant areas of the individual's everyday life and to initiate ways to alter these beliefs and their subsequent behaviors. Often, a detailed examination of these beliefs is carried out by looking at the way the patient distorts the therapist (transference) to satisfy powerful, yet unacknowledged, needs. The patient may idealize the therapist and rely excessively on his or her responses. Or the patient may reveal a distrust of the therapist under a pretense of cooperation. Dreams about the therapist may belie how the therapist is being used as a replacement (transference object) for a significant person in childhood who helped determine the patient's sense of worth.

Many patients will not develop grossly distorted views of the therapist that recapitulate earlier relationships but will reveal the inappropriate remnants of childhood belief systems in their relationships with others. As patients describe their interaction with spouses, colleagues, and other emotionally relevant individuals, the irrational fears, demands, and self-judgments that emerge are distinguished from more appropriate concerns and conflicts.

In a similar manner, unrealistic self-inhibitions along with anxieties over gratifications and masochistic self-reproaches are scrutinized to reveal their historical, maladaptive function. (With each discovery, the patient will use the resulting information in the service of change.) As the patient's repertoire of behavior enlarges, new experiences are reported that form the basis of further analysis. The goal is for the patient to base his or her estimation of self and others on realistic, adult criteria rather than on the carryovers from the distant past, which created the vulnerability to depression.

Ongoing Treatment

Depression is a recurrent illness, and maintenance drug therapy is often necessary. As in the earlier phases of combined treatment, psychotherapeutic communication may be employed to encourage patients to continue their medication, even in the face of ongoing side effects. This is not a minor function of psychotherapy. As patients gain in strength, and the last depressive episode recedes from memory, there is a natural wish to assume that no future depressions will develop. If antidepressant (or lithium) treatment is producing side effects, as is common, many patients will wish to discontinue their medications. The psychiatrist must summon the memory of the alliance during the acute phases of the past depressive illness to discourage premature drug discontinuation. In fact, encouraging the continuation of maintenance medication underlines the importance of establishing and maintaining an empathic therapeutic alliance. The patient must trust the psychiatrist's understanding and appraisal of the recent illness and rely on the psychiatrist's judgment about continuing medication, because the patient's own judgment may be compromised by defense mechanisms of denial or repression of the severity of the depression.

During this phase of maintenance antidepressant drug treatment, the psychiatrist's own bias about the role of drugs in psychiatric treatment may be tested. For some psychiatrists, the use of drugs is the primary therapeutic modality that is available for depression, and an ongoing psychotherapeutic relationship may be unnecessary, inefficient, and even destructive to the patient's growing sense of autonomy. For others, the use of drugs is a sign of empathic psychotherapeutic failure, and the sooner drugs are discontinued, the sooner "real therapy," i.e., psychotherapy, can begin. Such therapists may see the ongoing use of drugs as interfering with psychological explorations and the associative process because specific information regarding dose, side effects, and symptom response must be obtained.

It is our impression that most psychiatrists now recognize the importance of dual psychopharmacology-psychotherapeutic approaches to the patient who has recovered from a depression, but who may continue to be vulnerable to future depressions. Some psychiatrists at this recovery phase may even use the psychotherapeutic relationship to educate the patient about depressions, and teach them to recognize the early warning signs, so that reinstitution of antidepressant medication or adjustment of antidepressant dosages can take place. Others, however, may use the medication as part of the therapeutic process itself.

Psychotherapy may well continue even after the patient has altered his or her inner world and external behavior toward a more fulfilling and resilient adaptation. Others in the patient's close environment, although not wishing a depressive relapse, may attempt (often unconsciously) to undo the changes that have been achieved and to have the patient return to his or her earlier familiar, if more pathogenic, mode of being. The patient may need the therapist to aid in his or her resolve to perpetuate the newly acquired sense of self, despite external opposition. Therapy usually ends gradually as the individual has anchored his or her altered sense of self in a reality that allows for a life that offers a greater measure of satisfaction and meaning.

CASE EXAMPLES

The following case examples illustrate the benefits and hazards of combining pharmacotherapy and psychotherapy. Cases have been selected that illustrate the benefits and problems that arise when both therapies are administered by the same person; others have been selected to illustrate the benefits and risks of having pharmacotherapy and psychotherapy administered by two different care providers.

Miss A—Successful Combination of Pharmacotherapy and Psychotherapy; Therapist and Prescriber Are the Same Person

There may be patients for whom the prescribing psychopharmacologist naturally and easily also becomes the psychotherapist. There may also be clinical situations in which the psychotherapist, in the course of psychotherapeutic treatment, may prescribe drugs for the treatment of a depression, without jeopardizing the psychotherapy. Clinical experience as illustrated by this case suggests that, in some cases, the combined role of prescriber and therapist serves to augment both aspects of treatment leading to a successful outcome. This case also illustrates a common clinical situation— during the course of psychotherapy, prescription of antidepressants may result in symptomatic reduction and enhancement of the psychotherapy.

Miss A, a 20-year-old college dropout, entered psychotherapy because of fear of close relationships with men, an inability to attend to scholastic work despite considerable intellectual gifts, and estrangement from her parents. Although unhappy, she did not appear clinically depressed during the 1st year of her treatment. During this time in psychotherapy, she described emotionally unavailable although caring parents and a lifelong sense of unworthiness. She was unaware of ever having been depressed or angry. Rather, she considered her difficulties as her own failure to live up to the standards set by her perfectionistic and successful parents. Her awareness of her intellectual abilities only made her feel more guilty and more unworthy.

During the 1st year of psychotherapy, Miss A underwent several major stresses. Difficulties with roommates followed problems with boyfriends, and she found herself increasingly alone. Her parents, although attentive and concerned, did not understand her unhappiness and were unsupportive. She was ambivalent about returning to school. Unhappiness increased, and it became apparent that her symptoms were now those of a major depression. Her sleep was interrupted, her appetite dulled, and her energy almost nonexistent. Although she faithfully came to psychotherapy appointments, she would sometimes sit quietly, sadly, and tearfully, not able to talk or to verbalize her feelings.

The psychotherapist, recognizing the symptoms of major depression and concerned about her worsening life circumstances and her inability to use her psychotherapy sessions, began antidepressant treatment. Her response was rapid and gratifying. As her sleep, appetite, and energy improved, so did her outlook and her participation in the psychotherapy. Her sessions became more animated and more associative. For the first time, she became able to express negative feelings for her parents and even to acknowledge anger. Although still unhappy, she was no longer depressed.

Miss A illustrates the ideal result of combining psychotherapy and psychopharmacology. Although the former treatment was the treatment of choice for her to grow psychologically independent from her parents and to restructure her self-image, it is apparent that the psychotherapy could not have proceeded without therapeutic antidepressant drug treatment.

Although Miss A illustrates the introduction of drug therapy into a psychotherapy, the reverse process also may occur: psychotherapy can be started in the context of ongoing drug treatment. Some patients who are suffering from a symptomatic depression and who seek pharmacologic treatment may become aware of long-standing psychological conflict that may have contributed to the development of a depression. Such patients may wish to enter psychotherapy even though their depressive symptoms have been successfully treated with drugs. Consider the case of Mrs. B.

Mrs. B—Psychotherapy Begins in the Context of Successful Pharmacotherapy

Mrs. B, thrice married, entered therapy because of the irrational conviction that her third husband was having affairs with women who worked in his office. Despite all reassurances to the contrary, she described elaborate trysts that might conceivably occur when he was away on business. She admitted that her worries were irrational, but they were persistent.

Mrs. B had been severely sexually abused as a child and had often felt degraded or disregarded in her two prior marriages. Despite professional success, her accomplishments only reinforced her belief that her husbands did not care for her, because she was defective and unworthy. Her present husband, unlike the others, genuinely loved her, was extremely faithful and attentive, and was very perplexed by her concern for his fidelity.

Mrs. B came to her initial psychiatric appointments suffering from symptoms of major depression of moderate severity. Vegetative signs, low self-esteem, and depressed affect were all obvious. She had not considered psychotherapy because previous therapeutic experiences had left her feeling empty and angry.

Antidepressant drugs were started, and Mrs. B soon felt more energetic and optimistic. Nevertheless, her obsessive worries persisted, and she attempted to accompany her husband on business trips whenever possible. As this soon became impractical, she recontacted the prescribing psychiatrist and requested psychotherapy. She did not wish a new therapist; she trusted the doctor who had prescribed her drugs and relieved her symptomatic distress, and who knew her history.

As antidepressant medication continued, Mrs. B began to discuss, for the first time, the abuse she had suffered as a child. Her affective response to these long-repressed memories was nearly overwhelming, and she frequently expressed gratitude that her therapist was capable of understanding the need for symptom-relieving medication, should that need arise. The dual role of physician-therapist apparently provided enough reassurance to allow the painful reconstruction of past traumas to unfold.

For many patients, a physician as caregiver retains a special power of understanding and comfort. The ability to diagnose illness and to successfully treat it with medications may, for these patients, serve as a concrete illustration of the physician's caring. The administration of medication that eases pain reinforces this trust and cements a therapeutic alliance. How many of us do not trust and care for a doctor who has understood our suffering, correctly diagnosed its cause, and successfully treated it? In the context of such a strong trust, the psychotherapy may rapidly and successfully proceed. Psychotherapists who are adept at using medications, therefore, may find their therapeutic work enhanced by the judicious use of medications.

The cases of Miss A and Mrs. B illustrate the natural transition from a single therapeutic approach into the combined approach by one caregiver. The introduction of this second treatment approach may require a shift in style of interaction between treater and patient. For example, in the normal course of work, a pharmacologist may be highly interactive, medically oriented, and reassuring with a depressed patient who is receiving medication. Such a style, however, may be inappropriate during traditional psychodynamic psychotherapy. If a psychopharmacologist is to begin psychotherapy, a shift in style may be necessary. Alternatively, a reflective and relatively noninteractive psychotherapist may need to become more active, more questioning, and more medically oriented if medications are to be prescribed during the course of psychotherapy. For some patients, such a shift in the doctor's style is unsettling and countertherapeutic and may reinforce a decision not to enter psychotherapy.

Mr. C—The Patient Who Didn't Want Psychotherapy: Drugs Leading to Combined Treatment

Mr. C, a 51-year-old professional man, considered himself logical and fully in control of his life and emotions. When he became clinically depressed, he attempted to understand the genesis of his disorder by reading a considerable body of lay and professional literature concerning depression. His own diagnosis of his symptom pattern was correct: he was suffering from a major depressive disorder. Despite a stormy marriage and ambivalent feelings about his professional status, he insisted that his symptoms were entirely due to a familial tendency to depression (from his mother, who had been clinically depressed several times during her life) and without relationship to current stresses in his life. His own view was of depression as an entirely medical illness, secondary to biochemical disarrangement within the central nervous system, and that antidepressant medications were the solution.

Mr. C began on a course of antidepressant medications, which rapidly cleared his vegetative symptoms. His energy, outlook, appetite, and sense of humor returned, and he was once again productive. However, stress in his marriage continued, and as his symptoms resolved, his wife now felt that she could initiate a separation. Despite his renewed work productivity, he also continued to question his choice of a profession and his commitment to a job that did not interest him, despite his success. Consequently, although the classic symptoms of depression had significantly, although not entirely, improved, he was left with a residual dysphoric emotional state that interfered with his ability to fully realize his potentials, or to enjoy his life. He grew sarcastic, irritable, petulant, and morose. There was a return of his questioning the meaning of his existence and a recurrence of the experience of hopelessness, helplessness, and worthlessness. However, his energy, sleep, appetite, and libido all continued to be excellent, and he neither appeared depressed nor admitted to a recurrence of his former depressive affect. In other words, he was unhappy, but not depressed.

At this point, approximately 6 months after the resolution of his depression, he began to express a wish to speak with the prescribing psychiatrist more frequently. He still denied the merit of psychotherapy and often tried to debate the psychiatrist about the validity of the psychotherapeutic approach. Although he acknowledged that his marital and professional predicaments were consistent with emotional and behavioral experiences that had occurred in earlier life, he also doubted their relevance to his current emotional upset. Nevertheless, he continued to seek out his psychiatrist and continued to discuss both his present and his past unhappiness, and their relationship to his current marital and professional predicaments.

Mr. C and his psychiatrist agreed to continue medication because of the possibility of relapse during this period of unhappy crisis. However, the psychiatrist grew increasingly aware that Mr. C was using their sessions together as psychotherapy without actually asking for a psychotherapeutic relationship. It was suggested that Mr. C formally enter into psychotherapy, while continuing his antidepressant medication, to which Mr. C agreed. However, the relationship between Mr. C and the psychiatrist had been defined for the entire 6 months of treatment as psychopharmacologic and medical in nature. In this relationship, the psychiatrist had been very active, had asked and answered many questions, had obtained frequent blood tests, and had entirely focused on the patient's somatic functioning. The psychiatrist did not feel comfortable "changing gears" and becoming less responsive to the patient's questions, less active in their discussions, and more inquiring of the patient's inner emotional conflict. In other words, the psychiatrist, having felt more of a physician during the pharmacological treatment, now did not feel comfortable becoming a nonmedical therapist. Mr. C agreed to meet with a new therapist, specifically for therapy. The separation of roles made it possible for the prescribing psychiatrist to continue to carefully evaluate the pharmacological treatment without feeling confused about his role as therapist; he could ask and answer questions without concern that the transference relationship that is necessary for psychotherapy to proceed might be compromised.

Although it may be desirable for a psychopharmacologist to also serve as a psychotherapist, the case of Mr. C illustrates the usefulness of creating a split in the two functions. If the prescribing physician had initially been defined as therapist as well as drug prescriber, then the dual role could have been undertaken. However, because the request for psychotherapy came later into the relationship between doctor and patient, when both interacted with nonpsychotherapeutic behaviors, a switch into psychotherapy for both parties was difficult. Indeed, the psychiatrist recognized that it would be difficult for him to retreat from the more active role of drug prescriber to the reflective and more passive role of therapist, and that psychotherapy might be jeopardized.

For some depressed patients, any dynamic psychotherapy is not possible even with a separate therapist. These patients may be too threatened by increased self-awareness or confrontation with painful affect to sustain an ongoing psychotherapeutic relationship. For such patients, psychopharmacologic relief of depressive symptoms constitutes successful treatment, as illustrated in the following two case examples.

Ms. D—The Patient Who Didn't Want Psychotherapy: Drugs Reinforce Treatment Resistance

Ms. D presented with a severe depression complicated by marked melancholic features and continuous ruminations. The latter symptoms concerned a job position that Ms. D had accepted and that she now felt to have been a mistake. She constantly obsessed over having made an error in her career or that her life was a continual misery. She filled the early sessions with self-recriminations over being so stupid or short-sighted to have accepted her current job. She dated the onset of her depression to her discovery of this terrible mistake in judgment. After 2 weeks on tricyclic antidepressants, the patient was much improved; she was now able to sleep, had regained her appetite, had more energy, and was able to concentrate. She no longer reproached herself and decided that she would "stick out" the job for the extent of her contract and then seek other employment. Her depression had also mobilized her family to rally around her and offer her a good deal of nurturance and support. At this point, she refused to look at the possibility of having made the wrong decision and that this mistake had, in fact, precipitated a clinical depression. She thanked her doctor for his help but stated that as she was now recovered, she could see no point in stirring things up and was content to be seen for medication only. She emphasized that if she wished to confide anything about herself, she would do so with her family and not with an outsider.

This woman appeared to be threatened by what she might discover about herself and might have had such high standards for her behavior that therapy was simply too frightening a prospect.

Ms. E—Successful Drug Treatment May Be Sufficient; Psychotherapy May Be Toxic

Ms. E demonstrates a different yet related type of obstacle to psychotherapy. This patient also came for treatment in the midst of a severe clinical depression that also resolved with medication. However, as she began to discuss the reasons for her current depression (a feeling of not measuring up to the expectations of her superiors at work), she also started to recall incidents from her childhood that were extremely painful. The recollections were psychologically related to her current situation but elicited intolerable grief, sadness, and despair. These memories emerged spontaneously in the therapeutic setting without deliberate provocation. The result was that even on medication, the patient found the sessions too painful to endure and lived in dread of seeing her therapist. She decided that she could not endure the anxiety and torment that her therapy generated and asked to be seen (by another psychiatrist) for medication only. In this case, the therapeutic setting, or possibly some characteristic of the therapist, awakened terrifying memories that could not be contained or interpreted.

For most patients, however, medication enhances rather than limits the use of psychotherapy. Many individuals feel more secure in exploring painful or possibly depressive experiences with the assurance that medication will protect them from reexperiencing the severe depression that consideration of such topics might have caused in the past. Some discomfort is an inherent part of honestly looking at oneself and one's past but, in vulnerable individuals, medication can prevent the escalation of this necessary dysphoria into clinical depression.

Some patients are treated in psychotherapy either by nonphysician therapists or by psychiatrists who do not wish to prescribe medications in the course of their psychotherapeutic treatment. When antidepressant medications are indicated, patients of these therapists commonly are referred to a psychopharmacologist so that treatment becomes divided between two caregivers. This split in caregiving may be therapeutically beneficial for some patients. For example, the psychotherapist need not alter interactive style with the patient, nor does the patient need to see the therapist in a new role. The psychotherapy may continue unchanged and the prescription of an antidepressant can be defined by both patient and therapist as "going to the doctor." When there is cooperation, mutual respect, and open communication between the two caregivers, such divided care may be extremely beneficial for the depressed patient, as illustrated by Mrs. F.

Mrs. F—Therapist and Prescriber Are Different: Successful Outcome

Mrs. F, a 63-year-old woman, had lived for many years with a philandering and inattentive husband. Having no profession or postcollege training, she found herself without meaningful activity after her children were grown and had left home.

Although she was not in financial need, she began to buy property, renovate it, and sell it at a profit, and, within a few years, she became exceedingly successful, wealthy, and financially independent from her husband. He grew more estranged from her as her independence increased, and finally left her for a young woman. Mrs. F became acutely depressed, with severe vegetative symptoms, hopelessness, helplessness, worthlessness, and suicidal thoughts. She entered psychotherapy and for the first time in her life began to focus on her inner emotional experience.

Her therapist helped her to realize that she was furious at her husband and had been angry for many years of the marriage. Always raised to be dutiful and respectful of one's husband, and always honoring her distinguished, patrician father, she had never considered the validity of her own anger.

As her therapy progressed, however, her depressive symptoms only worsened. She experienced her new emotional awareness as a burden and as evidence of her guilt at not having been forgiving enough of her husband's indiscretions. The more she exposed her emotions, and the more she became aware of them, the more depressed she became. However, her therapeutic work soon changed from historical inquiry and emotional exposure to obsessive self-doubt and self-blame for her predicament. She was unable to discuss her past, except to castigate herself for not being a good-enough wife, mother, and even daughter. She saw herself as always depressed, never "good enough," and useless. Long periods of silence would develop during the psychotherapy sessions, which the patient characterized as not having anything worthwhile to say. She began to wonder if she were wasting the therapist's valuable treatment time, which could be better spent with another more deserving patient.

The therapist referred the patient for a psychopharmacology consultation with the following questions: Is this patient's depression biological? Since there are clear psychological precipitants, would antidepressants be helpful? Would the use of antidepressants inhibit the progress of emotional unfolding in the therapy?

At the time of the consultation, the patient was severely depressed, had lost 12 pounds, was hardly sleeping, and was nonfunctional in her real estate work. She was unable to drive a car by herself, and her grown children were preparing her food and taking her to her therapy appointments. She was haggard, relatively unkempt, and enormously sad, exuding a sense of hopelessness. She had lost her husband, her work, and now had nothing but an unbearable dependence on her children, which only made her feel more guilty and more depressed.

The patient was hospitalized and started on a tricyclic antidepressant. Within 2 weeks, she had begun to sleep and eat well and was discharged to outpatient treatment. She continued to see her therapist and to make regular visits to her prescribing psychiatrist. In psychotherapy, she now had more energy and was no longer hopeless. Although still unhappy, she was able to appraise her current life crisis more objectively and appreciate that she was not totally to blame for the dissolution of her marriage. She had only minor side effects from her antidepressants and willingly continued the prescription. The therapist and the prescribing physician maintained regular, frequent contact with each other to discuss the patient's mental status and her ability to use psychotherapy. After 1 month of combined treatment, the patient's depressive symptoms had nearly vanished. She had gained weight and evidenced improved grooming and more energy and began to plan to reopen her real estate office. In psychotherapy, she now talked animately about her depression and anger and recognized that she had experienced previous depressive episodes, but had mistaken them for "inadequacy, boredom, and uselessness."

The patient resumed her former life and continued active psychotherapy, which she now described as liberating. She described patterns of relationships with men, based on the relationship with her father, and realized the self-perpetuating nature of her dependence and her anger at men. She continued her medication for 6 months and then gradually tapered the dose, under supervision of the prescribing physician. Psychotherapy continued, and the patient has remained free from depression for 2 years.

Mrs. F illustrates the difficulty of conducting meaningful psychotherapeutic work during a severe major depression. Not only is there an inhibition of both mental and physical energy necessary to engage in psychotherapeutic work, but the depressed patient may only use the experience to further support his or her own depressed, negative self-image. Every past experience is interpreted as further evidence of failure of character, failure in life. The therapist may become frustrated, and the patient then concludes that he or she is a failure in therapy as well.

Therapists who work with depressed patients may misinterpret the content of psychotherapeutic sessions. Confession, self-revelation, and assuming responsibility for life's problems may be thought of as signs of psychological growth and maturity rather than as depressive symptoms. This is especially true in patients like Mrs. F, who have not led a life of inward self-examination, and for whom each early therapy session may seem like a revelation. For depressed patients, however, the appearance of assuming responsibility for one's life (as opposed to projecting or displacing blame on others) may be an inappropriate or exaggerated assumption of blame arising out of a depressive self-loathing. Such patients may begin to see all of the problems during the course of a lifetime as due to their failures, weaknesses, etc. This erroneous and exaggerated self-blame can be reinforced by a well-meaning therapist who attempts to "be in touch with" the patient's feelings. The patient's emotional state may be regarded as appropriate and consonant with the material being discussed in the therapy sessions and not seen as markedly colored and distorted by depressive illness.

In the case of Mrs. F, both the therapist and prescribing physician agreed on the presence of a depression, and both agreed on the need for drug treatment. The therapist did not see the use of drugs as a sign that therapy had failed, i.e., that either she had failed as the therapist, or that the patient had failed in her role. The physician did not regard the therapy as a failure, or as a mistake. Rather, both therapist and physician formed a communicative partnership that focused on the patient's current mental status. The therapist strongly encouraged (actually insisted) on the psychopharmacology consultation and also strongly supported the period of brief hospitalization for institution of drug treatment. Without this support, drug treatment would not have been possible. The prescribing physician strongly encouraged the patient to remain in a psychotherapeutic relationship so that therapeutic work could continue when the depression's severity lifted. Both therapist and prescriber emphasized the need for both approaches and supported each other to the patient and in weekly communication (more frequently during the hospitalization). The patient's experience of this bilateral support was one of a solid framework of professional help. She commented that she felt safe and reassured by the bilateral approach and confident in the treatment decisions. Many months after the depression had lifted, she commented that she would not have been able to take the drugs or agree to hospitalization without the support of the therapist. She also commented that she would not be able to continue in psychotherapy without the knowledge that her therapist would be able to recognize a depression, should it develop, and refer her to the prescribing physician for another course of drug treatment. The presence of the bilateral treatment was critical for the progress in this patient's psychological health.

When the therapist and prescriber are different persons, there is an increased likelihood of conflict and therapeutic failure. The patient and psychotherapist may share a view that the drug prescriber is an alien intruder into the therapeutic alliance and relationship. Or, the prescriber and the patient may view the therapist as having failed therapeutically, or as having missed a diagnosis. Or, the patient may shift alliances between therapist and prescriber, alternating allegiance first with one, then with the other, making coherent treatment nearly impossible. Under such circumstances, either the psychotherapy may fail, as illustrated by Mr. G, or the pharmacotherapy may fail, as illustrated by Mrs. H.

Mr. G—Therapist-Prescriber Split: Unsuccessful Resolution—Psychotherapy Fails

Mr. G, a 38-year-old student, had been in psychotherapy for many years. His treatment focused on a chronic difficulty establishing durable relationships with women, and also on establishing a durable professional identity. The child of an overbearing father and a passive but controlling mother, Mr. G worked at jobs that were unfulfilling and established liaisons with inappropriate women. He liked his psychotherapist, who was extremely supportive, available, and paternal.

Mr. G's psychological problems seemed intractable, and he grew despondent, withdrawn, anergic, and suicidal. Fearing the development of a major depression, his therapist started treatment with an antidepressant drug. Severe side effects developed, without any relief of symptoms. The psychotherapist became increasingly preoccupied with the search for an appropriate medication, and less psychotherapeutically active. Mr. G perceived this change in his therapist first as a loss of interest, and then as an abandonment. He discontinued his medication and terminated his psychotherapy. Mr. G illustrates the hazard of a change in role by the caregiver. When a psychotherapist of long duration changes roles and becomes a psychopharmacologist, or vice versa, the patient may react by feeling abandoned. Not infrequently, the patient then becomes furious (transference rage) and ends the relationship. Alternatively, patients in this situation perceive themselves as hopeless, again in a transference context (my parents really don't love me because I am worthless/hopeless/defective/unlovable), and feel worse. Fortunately, Mr. G sought out consultation, which recommended continued psychotherapy rather than continued pharmacotherapy, and a new and more successful therapeutic alliance was initiated.

Mrs. H—Therapist-Prescriber Split: Unsuccessful Resolution—Pharmacotherapy Fails

Mrs. H is a 40-year-old, very successful executive, who is married and a mother. She entered psychotherapy, with a nonphysician, because of the threatened breakup of her marriage. As psychotherapy proceeded, she became aware of long-standing behavior patterns that were self-destructive and that contributed to the marital difficulties. She also became aware of her ambivalence about being independent and her hidden need to rely on a man toward whom she could feel enraged. In the course of her psychotherapy, she became clinically depressed and was sent for psychopharmacology consultation.

Mrs. H was indeed depressed, although only moderately so. Antidepressant drugs were considered to be potentially helpful and were recommended. The patient wished for a drug trial, but the therapist objected, concerned that medications might either mask the emergence of the patient's depressive affect, which had been so laboriously nurtured through psychotherapy, or that the patient would see the use of medications as another route to avoid self-awareness. Despite numerous discussions between therapist and prescriber, and a period of further therapy without drug treatment during which the patient remained depressed, there was no agreement on the proper clinical course. The patient, feeling torn between the two caregivers, discontinued contact with the psychopharmacologist. She noted that her psychotherapeutic relationship was dear to her, and that her therapist knew her best, accepted her with all her faults (including her depression), and would see her through.

Perhaps a depression of greater severity would have resolved this intertreater conflict. Perhaps the conflict between the two caregivers was, in part, fostered by an ambivalence in the patient herself, reflecting her own need to divide others into good and bad objects. The therapist was all good, all caring. The pharmacologist, who might have been good, had to be made bad, and become the target for the negative transference affects that could not be expressed toward the psychotherapist. Psychopharmacologists must be aware of this possibility when they offer medications in the context of psychotherapy with another person. Alternatively, the split may develop in the opposite direction. The therapist is seen as impotent, uncaring, and abandoning, in contrast to the prescribing psychopharmacologist, who becomes invested with the magical, curative, and nurturing powers. Such a split, in either direction, is destructive.

Therapists and pharmacologists must remain aware of such a potential for inappropriate affects to be directed either toward them or away from them toward the other caregiver. When a patient is criticizing the other care provider, then one must not reinforce such a split and projection by disparaging the therapeutic strategies, techniques, or goals of the other treater. Open therapeutic discussion of any tendency to split people into good and bad and then to direct opposing affects toward these split objects is essential. Equally important, if a shared therapeutic program is to be effective, is open communication between therapist and pharmacologist, and each must be able to reality test these projected affects from the patient.

CONCLUSION

Psychopharmacology and psychotherapy may produce therapeutic effects, via different mechanisms, in different patient populations. For patients who are concretely oriented in the medical model (and for like-minded psychiatrists), pharmacologic antidepressant relief of major depressive symptoms represents adequate and complete treatment. Psychotherapeutic communication for such patients probably is limited to encouragement of drug-taking behavior, reassurance, and enhancement of coping strategies that can be used when the patient is no longer depressed.

At the other end of the patient spectrum, psychologically minded patients (and like-minded psychotherapists) may see the depression as rooted in a complex biological-psychological matrix. Although not denying the importance of the biological dysfunction that is associated with depression, and the need for pharmacological readjustment of such dysfunction, these patients and their psychiatrists believe that psychological character formation, childhood and prior experience, and current life stresses all play a role in the patient's evaluation of their place in the world, their value as a person, and their ability to work, love, and fulfill a potential that is accurately assessed. Depression is understood as a symptom of such psychological dysfunction, perhaps rooted in biological and genetic vulnerability, but nevertheless influenced by one's interaction with the world and the people who inhabit it. For these people, therapy not only consists of symptom reduction, but an identification and strengthening of those inner aspects of personal experience that are believed to contribute to depression. The taking of an antidepressant drug is seen as the beginning of a treatment program, rather than the entire program per se.

It is our impression, however, that most patients, as well as most psychiatrists and psychotherapists, understand depression and the unhappiness that may accompany depression as a complex interaction of psychological and biological variables. Psychotherapy is seen as facilitating psychopharmacological treatment of depression, and psychopharmacology is understood as paving the way toward energizing the process of psychotherapy.

Regardless of the personal orientation of the patient, and the theoretical bias of the psychiatrist-therapist, several factors must operate for successful treatment of a depression to occur. Most important, there must be an alliance between patient and healer that facilitates the treatment program. The development of a therapeutic alliance, whether it centers around drugs or around psychotherapy, or around both, requires the careful, gradual establishment of trust between two human beings who may start out as strangers, and between whom power and potency is unequal. The depressed patient, of all psychiatric patients, may feel helpless, hopeless, and worthless, especially in the presence of a healer who is seen as competent, self-assured, and potent. The development of the alliance requires trust on the part of the patient and patience on the part of the healer, and both must develop in the context of symptoms that may be severely compromising the patient's usual coping abilities and physical and mental skills.

It is our opinion that most patients who are depressed benefit from both the pharmacological and the psychological approach to treatment. As we have suggested, during the acute, severely symptomatic phases of the depression, psychotherapy may not be possible, and healing efforts should be directed toward symptom relief, assessment of the patient's progress, and careful building of the therapeutic alliance. As the patient becomes less symptomatic, gradual psychotherapeutic exploration may be possible. With the elimination of depressive symptoms, psychologically minded patients may find the motivation, energy, and enthusiasm to enter into psychotherapy, as part of the continued treatment of the depressive episode, and to restructure and repair inner functioning so as to prevent or mitigate future depressions.

REFERENCES

Akiskal HS: Dysthymic disorder: psychopathology of proposed chronic depressive subtypes. Am J Psychiatry 140:11–20, 1983

American Psychiatric Association: Diagnostic and Statistical Manual of Mental Disorders, 3rd Edition, Revised. Washington, DC, American Psychiatric Association, 1987

Brown GW, Harris TO: Social Origins of Depression. London, Tavistock, 1978

Keller MB, Shapiro RW: "Double depression": superimposition of acute depressive episodes on chronic depressive disorder. Am J Psychiatry 139:438–442, 1982

Ostow M: Drugs in Psychoanalysis and Psychotherapy. New York, Basic Books, 1962

Scott J: Chronic depression. Br J Psychiatry 153:287–297, 1988

Afterword

It may be useful for us to summarize briefly our impressions of what has emerged from this review of combined treatment of depression and provide some of our conclusions and clinical recommendations.

In Chapter 1, we reviewed the 17 studies available in the literature that have compared the combination of psychotherapy and pharmacotherapy with either alone. We conclude that combined therapy is no less effective than either treatment alone and that concerns about negative interaction are unfounded. On most measures in most studies, the effect of combined therapy equals either psychotherapy or pharmacotherapy alone, whereas on some measures in some studies, the combination shows some superiority. If there is an edge to combined treatment versus psychotherapy alone it is in faster onset in the treatment of somatic symptoms of depression. If there is an edge to the combination versus pharmacotherapy alone it is in interpersonal and cognitive functioning and the stability of remission. We discovered that the existing literature has many methodological problems that might lead to Type I and II errors.

Drs. Hollon, DeRubeis, and Evans addressed the clinical and conceptual design issues involved in combining tricyclic pharmacotherapy with individual cognitive therapy. They described their recently completed controlled clinical trial comparing imipramine versus cognitive therapy versus their combination with depressed, nonpsychotic, nonbipolar outpatients. They found that both single modalities were comparably effective in terms of acute response, with the combined modality being more effective still. At 2-year follow-up, cognitive therapy, whether initially provided alone or in combination with pharmacotherapy, evidenced a marked prophylactic effect in reducing relapse and recurrence.

Drs. Covi, Lipman, and Smith reported on two controlled trials studying the combination of group psychotherapy and pharmacotherapy. In both studies, they found marginal advantages to combined treatment and no difficulty combining group cognitive therapy with medication.

Drs. Weissman and Klerman discussed the results of their studies of interpersonal psychotherapy in combination with amitriptyline in which they found evidence for an additive effect of the two modalities. They found no indication in their results of a negative interaction between pharmacotherapy and psychotherapy. Superiority for combined therapy over pharmacotherapy or psychotherapy alone appeared in the areas of lower patient dropout rate, enhanced patient acceptance of treatment, and more rapid symptom reduction.

Drs. Frank and Kupfer and Ms. Levenson reported on the data from a continuation study of recurrent unipolar patients treated with combined interpersonal psychotherapy and imipramine in continuation therapy. Their results suggest that combined therapy shows advantages over single-modality treatment in reducing the risk of relapse and in increasing patient retention in therapy.

Drs. Salzman and Bemporad presented a number of useful clinical guidelines suggesting the indication for combined treatment and its likely effects.

It should, by now, be obvious that the available research findings in this area (as in most others as well) are sufficiently limited that many different plausible conclusions might be drawn. We cannot and do not claim any special currency for our own clinical approach but find that it has been useful in guiding us toward clinical indications for combined treatment. The variables that most influence our decision concerning whether to use combined treatment for depression are the severity, urgency, and chronicity of the patient's psychopathology, past treatment response, and the patient's preference. We will discuss these in turn.

We have found that there is a U-shaped relationship between our use of combined treatment and the severity of the patient's depression—i.e., we tend to withhold a combined approach from the least and most severe depressions and instead use combined treatment most often for the moderately severe cases. Our rationale for this approach is that many, if not most, milder depressions (particularly acute ones) respond quite well to psychotherapy delivered alone and do not warrant committing the patient to a long trial of antidepressant medication, which carries with it expense, inconvenience, side effects, and the risk of false attributions by the patient and/or the clinician that it was the medication, rather than the psychotherapy, that was curative. In these situations, we indicate to the patient that the type of depression he or she has is usually responsive to specific psychotherapeutic techniques and homework assignments. Medication is not used for the first weeks or months of treatment and is added later only if the depressive symptoms fail to remit or become worse or more urgent. This approach saves many patients what turn out to be unnecessary medication trials and makes clearer to all concerned what were the active ingredients promoting remission. This latter point is important in guiding the choice of subsequent treatments and also in providing the patient with a sense of self-mastery in having learned new ways of coping with and overcoming depression. Even when medication becomes necessary, it is important to continue the psychotherapy, which may become more effective when delivered adjunctly. A positive drug response often helps the patient to participate more fruitfully in psychotherapy. Psychotherapy may also help to reduce relapse when the drug is eventually withdrawn and may have a prophylactic effect in reducing the risk of subsequent recurrences.

Those patients who present with the most severe depressions generally require hospitalization and are often unable to participate in any psychotherapy beyond that provided by general support and a caring physician's attitude. Very severely depressed individuals may even experience attempts at psychotherapy as unduly stressful and become even more hopeless and guilty because of their inability to participate. The first-line treatment for such patients should be somatic—i.e., medication or electroconvulsive therapy—and psychotherapy should be added only when patients have recovered sufficiently to engage in it.

Thus, for patients with less severe depression, we generally recommend beginning with psychotherapy alone and adding medication later and only if needed. For the most severely affected patients, we begin with somatic treatment alone and add psychotherapy only after they have responded. It is for patients midway between these levels of severity that combined treatment may be selected as a first-line approach. Such individuals are experiencing sufficiently severe suicidal ideation, somatic discomfort, and/or inability to function that it appears clinically unwise to begin psychotherapy alone, but they are sufficiently engageable that it is feasible to combine psychotherapy with drug treatment. This can usually be done on an outpatient basis, but combined treatment can also be begun in the hospital for those patients who are sufficiently suicidal, noncompliant, or physically ill as to make hospitalization necessary. In our experience, there are several other hints that combined treatment may be the preferred first line of approach. The best predictor is likely to be the patient's previous treatment response. If combined treatment has worked before, or if psychotherapy or medication has been by itself only partially helpful before, it may be wise to try both treatments together. The course of the patient's disorder may also be important in the decision to select combined treatments. We have found that chronic depressions are more likely to require combined treatment.

For many patients, various alternative approaches — alone and together — may all seem plausible. It is often useful to describe these options to the patient, indicate their possible advantages and disadvantages, and then let the patient choose among them. This sharing with the patient the responsibility for treatment chosen is likely to increase the level of cooperation and active participation.

These are largely unsupported clinical guidelines, and it is clear that much additional research remains to be done before we will have widely accepted and more precise indications for recommending combined treatment. In the meantime, we should feel fortunate that there are so many different effective ways of treating depression and that these seem to go well with one another. This affords us the opportunity of matching our treatments to our patients' needs and preferences. We can thus feel confident that, given enough time and cooperation, we can almost always find a treatment or combination of treatments that will succeed in alleviating and perhaps preventing the great suffering and risk occasioned by depression.

—